GAMBLING AS AN ADDICTIVE BEHAVIOUR

Impaired Control, Harm Minimisation, Treatment and Prevention

"If thinking about addiction is going to change, the study of excessive gambling is likely to be one of the richest sources of new ideas" (Jim Orford). In this book, the authors present the most recent and evolving research into gambling, showing the psychological variables that govern the erosion or maintenance of self-control over gambling behaviour. These studies provide an empirical basis for a model of impaired control of gambling. Impaired control, in its broadest sense, is considered to be the defining psychological construct of all the addictive behaviours and occupies a central position in conceptualising the addictive aspects of gambling.

MARK DICKERSON is a Professor of Psychology at the University of Western Sydney, Sydney and JOHN O'CONNOR is a Consultant Psychologist, Senior Lecturer in the School of Medicine at Flinders University, Adelaide.

T0292115

INTERNATIONAL RESEARCH MONOGRAPHS IN THE ADDICTIONS (IRMA)

Series Editor
Professor Griffith Edwards
National Addiction Centre
Institute of Psychiatry, London

Volumes in this series present important research from major centres around the world on the basic sciences, both biological and behavioural, that have a bearing on the addictions. They also address the clinical and public health applications of such research. The series will cover alcohol, illicit drugs, psychotropics and tobacco. It is an important resource for clinicians, researchers and policy-makers.

Also in this series

Cannabis and Cognitive Functioning
Nadia Solowij
ISBN 0 521 159114 7

A Community Reinforcement Approach to Addiction Treatment
Robert J. Meyers and William R. Miller
ISBN 0 521 77107 2

Circles of Recovery: Self-Help Organizations for Addictions
Keith N. Humphreys
ISBN 0 521 79299 0

Alcohol and the Community: A Systems Approach to Prevention
Harold D. Holder
ISBN 0 521 59187 2

Treatment Matching in Alcoholism
Thomas F. Babor and Frances K. Del Boca
ISBN 0 521 65112 3

Cannabis Dependence: Its Nature, Consequences and Treatment
Roger A. Roffman and Robert S. Stephens
ISBN 0 521 81447 2

GAMBLING AS AN ADDICTIVE BEHAVIOUR

Impaired Control, Harm Minimisation, Treatment and Prevention

MARK DICKERSON
School of Psychology
University of Western Sydney, Sydney

JOHN O'CONNOR
School of Medicine
Flinders University, Adelaide

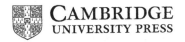
CAMBRIDGE
UNIVERSITY PRESS

CAMBRIDGE UNIVERSITY PRESS
Cambridge, New York, Melbourne, Madrid, Cape Town,
Singapore, São Paulo, Delhi, Tokyo, Mexico City

Cambridge University Press
The Edinburgh Building, Cambridge CB2 8RU, UK

Published in the United States of America by Cambridge University Press, New York

www.cambridge.org
Information on this title: www.cambridge.org/9780521399197

First published 2006
First paperback edition 2011

A catalogue record for this publication is available from the British Library

ISBN 978-0-521-84701-8 Hardback
ISBN 978-0-521-39919-7 Paperback

Contents

Preface

This monograph provided the opportunity to describe a programme of gambling research completed at the School of Psychology, University of Western Sydney and to discuss the results in the context of contemporary research into problem and pathological gambling. As the principal researchers were mainly very able and independent-minded doctoral students the "programme" was by no means a coherent, planned sequence. Nonetheless, in the context of ongoing personal research, other postgraduate projects and collaboration with other academic staff, the body of work completed over the past 5 years or so has made some inroads on the agenda outlined in Dickerson & Baron (2000): by studying regular gamblers to focus on the psychological processes that erode and maintain subjective self-control over gambling behaviour.

The Australian gambling context provided a unique research opportunity having, as it does, significant populations of men and women who regularly engage in continuous forms of gambling such as electronic gaming machine (EGM) play, off-course betting and casino table games: the debt owed to those players who volunteered is acknowledged and the gratitude expressed to them previously repeated here. Whether they were involved in surveys, qualitative interviews or experimental studies, the research was utterly dependent on their participation.

The evolution of the ideas and methods was often a direct function of the success of the individuals in the PhD programme, independent and responsive to advice rather than supervision, from founding member, now co-author (J. O'Connor), to John Haw, Andrew Kyngdon, Robyn Maddern, and still to complete, Morten Boyer and Lee Shepherd. This text would not have been possible without the results of their creativity and that of other postgraduates and colleagues. The twofold objective of bringing this work together has been to:

1. Challenge some of the empirical and theoretical assumptions about regular gamblers that have been used to underpin both the mental disorder, pathological gambling and related harm-prevention policy.

2. Illustrate common empirical ground between gambling and other addictive behaviours reaffirming common underlying psychological processes.

In reviewing the international context of problem gambling research the more usual sources such as refereed journals and new textbooks have been augmented by several reports describing national gambling reviews, for example in the USA, Australia and the UK. In addition, particularly in Australasia various state and federal government departments have been very active in funding research programmes into gambling and problem gambling. Typically university-based research teams following international competitive tendering have completed projects and the quality of the work has often been of a high standard. However, as the reports are often designed to satisfy government requirements and not a journal article length and style, the findings have not appeared in the academic literature. In this monograph we have followed the lead of other writers in the field who have referenced this body of work as it includes a number of important findings.

Declaration

During the period 1 July 1998 to 30 June 2003, I was employed by the University of Western Sydney (UWS) as the "Tattersall's Chair of Psychology", a professorial research appointment within the School of Psychology funded by Tattersall's. (Tattersall's is the largest privately owned business conglomerate in Australia whose core international business is lottery and gaming machine operations.) The position involved a competitive selection process in which Tattersall's was not involved. Tattersall's had naming rights only and if their financial support to the University had been withdrawn during the period of the contract the appointee remained on contract with UWS. Tattersall's provided no funding or support in kind for any of the School of Psychology research projects.

I am grateful to Tattersall's for providing the funding to my University that enabled me to focus entirely on research into gambling for the period of the contract.

I was appointed as a consultant to the Department of Human Services in Victoria from 1996 to 2003 advising on all aspects of research and policy relating to problem gambling: during the first 4 years I acted on behalf of UWS with payment going to the University and for the latter period was paid the fees as additional personal income.

Mark Dickerson
March 2005

At no time have I received funding from any of the gambling industries to fund research. On one occasion only I received an honorarium to write a short discussion article for an umbrella gambling industry body in which I expressed the opinion that it was not possible to suppress all developing forms of interactive (electronic) gambling and that strict legislative frameworks would be required to minimise likely harm.

John O'Connor
March 2005

Executive Summary

Chapter 1: Contemporary worldwide developments in the gambling industry and a brief historical comment provide the back-drop for an introduction to research into gambling and "pathological gambling". Definitions of the latter are discussed and international levels of prevalence are considered. Evidence is presented showing that men and women who gamble regularly (weekly or more often) on continuous forms of gambling (e.g. EGMs, casino table games, off-course betting) are most at risk of incurring harmful impacts arising from their gambling.

Chapter 2: The focus of the monograph, impaired self-control over gambling is defined and identified as a key psychological dependent variable in understanding pathological gambling and the harmful impacts of gambling. Two empirical research methodologies, traditional psychometric and mathematical psychology, for defining and measuring impaired self-control of gambling are described. Self-control over gambling is shown to be a central feature of regular gambling (a reliably measurable dimension, common to both regular gamblers and clinical cases of pathological gambling) that ranges from effortless control to extreme difficulty, despite repeated strenuous effort, to limit expenditure of time and money.

Chapter 3: A detailed review of the literature on problem gambling is presented, focusing on psychological variables that are likely to contribute to the erosion and/or maintenance of self-control over gambling. Variables reviewed include: current level of involvement in gambling, emotional factors, individual differences, alcohol consumption, cognitive variables and coping.

Chapter 4: Two recently completed empirical studies, one quantitative, one qualitative, identifying key psychological variables that contribute to the erosion of self-control over gambling are summarised, compared and contrasted.

Chapter 5: The implications for the psychological treatment of pathological gamblers, arising from the emerging model of impaired self-control over gambling, are discussed.

Chapter 6: The validity of the contemporary approach to harm minimisation, "responsible gambling", is challenged. In the context of the data showing how common, amongst ordinary regular gamblers, are reports of impaired self-control, it is argued that a totally new policy approach is required, one based on existing principles of consumer protection.

Chapter 7: A case study is presented of a single jurisdiction, Victoria in Australia, in which following the introduction of EGMs in the 1990s there developed an integrated set of harm minimisation strategies that have set international benchmarks. Data illustrating the efficacy of these over the past decade are presented. In the context of the arguments in the previous chapter the question arises whether the case study represents a public health success story, or a costly failure of policy selection.

Chapter 8: The research in measuring and modelling impaired control is critically evaluated. The essential nature of impaired control of gambling is described, and the implications and challenges for the "mental disorder" conceptualisation of pathological gambling are identified. The results are considered in the context of the addictive behaviours generally.

Glossary

EGM	Electronic gaming machine or "poker machine" common name in Australia (see gaming machines).
Excessive gambling	Indicates a level of involvement in gambling that encroaches on the resources allocated to other activities of daily life such as relationships and employment.
Expenditure	The net amount lost by gamblers, amount staked minus winnings.
Gambling	Staking or risking money on the outcome of uncertain future events driven mainly by chance; the most commonly legalised forms are betting on races and sports events, gaming machines, casino table games, keno and a variety of lotteries.
Gaming	All forms of gambling except wagering, that is betting on sports events and racing.
Gaming machines	Machines derived from the original mechanical "one armed bandit" where the outcomes are entirely chance determined or where the player can make skilful choices, for example in simulated card games: pay-outs very greatly from "gifts" to over a million dollars in some casinos.
Instant lottery	Sometimes known as "scratchies"; on purchasing a panel is rubbed to remove a covering film to reveal whether a prize has been won.
Keno	Electronic version of bingo where players purchase a set of numbers, winning if they match the first set of numbers selected at random during play.

Lotteries	Includes a variety of forms, lotto, pools and instant lotteries. Typically involves the purchase/selection of numbers which if match those selected at random at the date and time of the draw may win very large pay-outs.
Odds	Statistical estimates of winning/losing: in wagering may also determine the relationship between the amount staked and the size of the amount won.
Off-course betting	Facility for wagering on races (horses and dogs) and other sporting events: may be stand-alone venue or incorporated into a casino, hotel or social club.
Pathological gamblers	Gamblers who are described as preoccupied with gambling and also satisfy other diagnostic criteria specified in the *Diagnostic and Statistical Manual of Mental Disorders, 4th edition* (DSM-IV) of the American Psychiatric Association (1994).
Prevalence of problem gambling	An epidemiological estimate of the proportion of a specified population that are seriously adversely affected by their gambling: typically estimated by general population survey measures, "current" prevalence referring to reports of harmful impacts occurring during the last year.
Problem gambling	Sometimes used to describe a mid-point between social, harm-free gambling and pathological gambling: in this monograph used to indicate gamblers who are currently experiencing significant harmful impacts arising from their gambling.
Scratch lottery	See Instant lottery above.
Sports betting	Wagering on the outcome of a sports event, the result or outcomes within a smaller time frame such as the next wicket to fall, sinking the next putt, scoring the next goal, etc.
Wagering	Gambling on racing and sports events.

Foreword

Like gamblers who experience the mixed emotions of excitement, hope, regret and depression, reading the foregoing chapters has left me with mixed feelings of stimulation, dismay and reassurance. Let me try to unpick the tangle, starting with stimulation.

Stimulation

I am greatly stimulated by Dickerson and O'Connor's central idea of a continuum of control and choice over gambling (they acknowledge their debt to Heather et al.'s idea of impaired control over the consumption of alcohol). In place of diagnosing pathology, they draw on a variety of studies that they and their colleagues have carried out, including a qualitative study of limit setting amongst 16–24-year-old regular gamblers, which support the continuum of control concept. The dimension runs from "free effortless enjoyment", via the exertion of increasing effort to resist, to a position in which self-control can scarcely be maintained. The 12-item Scale of Gambling Choices that their group has developed for assessing control over gambling correlates highly with scores on the most commonly used measure of problem gambling – The South Oaks Gambling Screen – and with measures of greater gambling involvement, more time and money spent gambling, and the accumulation of higher debts.

That way of understanding the essence of problematic gambling represents an important shift that is bound to be controversial. It recognises the reality of difficult-to-control gambling whilst rejecting the idea of a diagnosable entity called "pathological gambling" or "compulsive gambling". It is possible to be "addicted" to gambling in the sense of being habitually engaged in, or attached or devoted to the activity to such an extent that it is difficult to disengage from it despite harms that it may be causing. In extreme form it can be devastatingly disabling to individuals who experience it and can turn upside down the lives of affected families. But it is on a continuum, with large proportions of gamblers, particularly machine gamblers, experiencing some degree of erosion of control and choice. One implication is that any attempt to draw a line between those who have a gambling problem and those who do not is bound to be arbitrary. That may be a problem for epidemiologists and for service planners and those who seek to influence them. But it is a problem that we live with in many areas of health and well-being, including the closely parallel topic of difficult-to-control alcohol consumption.

Although the authors wish to focus on erosion of self-control as candidate for being the core process in addiction, they recognise that it cannot easily be separated from the harmful impacts of uncontrolled gambling, since harm feeds a cycle of increasing impact and strength of attachment to the activity. That is important because it acknowledges the need for a developmental component in a full model of impaired control over an activity such as gambling. It is not just the learning of a habit that underlies the erosion of choice, but also the further processes that become overlaid on top of habitual activity. In *Excessive Appetites* (Orford, 2001), I argued that much of that overlay can be thought of as the consequences of conflict. Conflict develops between the motivation to engage in activity that is rewarded and has become habitual and the motivation to minimise the harms that habitual activity is giving rise to. The consequences of that conflict, which can include demoralisation, poor information processing, compulsive behaviour, and alterations of social role and social group, very often have the effect of introducing new motives for continued gambling, and fewer opportunities for reward from activities alternative to gambling.

One of the further strengths of Dickerson and O'Connor's formulation is their recognition and explication of the complex but crucial role of the flux of emotions surrounding gambling. That includes: dysphoric mood, either preceding or following excessive gambling; the role of hope after a stake is placed, and the role of anticipated regret in supporting continued gambling; the arousing, but sometimes calming, effects of gambling; and the central role of "chasing" as a cognitive–emotional–behavioural constellation that contributes to continuing to gamble and to a raising of stakes; plus the motivating effects of the "near-miss". One of the intriguing complexities of most, perhaps all, forms of appetitive behaviour that can become excessive or out-of-control is that they can enhance mood in ways that are both positively and negatively reinforcing. Cooper et al. (1995) contrasted the "enhancing" effect of alcohol in increasing positive emotion, and the "coping" or self-medicating effect of decreasing negative emotions. These were distinct, but in practice positively correlated, so that only minorities of people were pure enhancement drinkers or pure coping drinkers. Similarly, Lesieur and Rosenthal (1991) found evidence for "action-seeking" and "escape-seeking" motives for gambling. Others have considered the cycle of emotions associated with single consumption episodes. For example, Hsu (1990) found that women who experienced eating binges were likely to choose terms such as "anxious" or "tense" to describe their feelings before a binge, "depressed" at stages during a binge, and "guilty" and "exhausted" at the end of a binge cycle. A similar cycle of emotions surrounding shopping episodes has been described by women who feel out-of-control over shopping (Dittmar, 2004).

Dismay

My feelings of dismay are related to what this work tells us about the rapidity of technological change and innovation in gambling, and the creation of more continuous and ever more dangerous forms of gambling. We are reminded that the slot machine, perhaps rather like the hypodermic needle in relation to drug taking, has been with us for only a little more than a 100 years. The authors illustrate some of the ways in which modern gambling machines have become much more complex than they once were. In one, a sequence of eight responses to the machine is possible, including selecting the pay-line, bet multiplication, feature option and further gambles, in place of a sequence of only three responses in the case of older, simpler machines that were available until around 1970 (see also Parke and Griffiths, 2004; Dowling et al., 2005). One effect is likely to be a considerable enhancement of the "illusion of control" (Langer and Roth, 1975) which has been shown to encourage continued play and is found to be more strongly held by problem gamblers (Griffiths, 1995). It is interesting to note that the median age of the machines in one of the studies reviewed by Dickerson and O'Connor was only 9 months.

A great strength of much of the work collected together in this book is that it takes us right into the nitty gritty of machine gambling. Using the detailed tracking data that is now available, the reality of machine gambling is exposed. The example provided in Chapter 6 is graphic. Half-an-hour into a session a regular player, on average playing about a dozen games a minute, would have played getting on for 400 games. Dickerson and O'Connor argue that it is a strange entertainment product that faces the purchaser with such a rapid sequence of complex winning and losing outcomes. Although the cost per game may appear trivial (on average only 40 cents for regular players of machines in New South Wales where the maximum stake is A$10 per game), the per annum spend for regular players totals about $8000 on average. They calculate that the maximum loss per hour has risen from just over $5 in the early 1950s to around $500 in the mid-1990s. Evidence from Canada, cited by Dickerson and O'Connor, suggests that nearly a quarter of regular machine players may have gambling problems, and their own finding from Australia is that it is unusual for regular machine players not to experience some degree of impaired control of their gambling.

There seems truth in their statement regarding machine gambling:

... an apparently innocuous mechanical gambling device, is now permitted to be sold as an automated, rapid and emotionally distracting product of unlimited sequences in venues specially designed to heighten the focus on gambling (p. 119).

That makes the policy issue as much one of consumer protection as a public health issue. Is the gambling machine in its modern form unethical? Does it at the very least need to be significantly modified in order to maintain the standards that would be expected of any other entertainment product? How, under the conditions so graphically illustrated, can freedom of choice reasonably be preserved for people who play such machines?

Not that earlier generations of gambling machines were innocuous. Even in the inter-war years in Britain voices with experience were being raised against them. For example, in 1927 the Lord Chief Justice stated that the slot machine, "was a pest and a most mischievous pest, because it operates on the minds of young persons and corrupts them in their youth" (cited by Clapson, 1992, p. 88). In 1932 the Chief Constable of the Metropolitan Police told Parliament that, "By far the most troublesome form of gaming [in] recent years is the automatic gaming machine of the 'fruit' variety" (cited by Clapson, 1992, p. 85).

In Chapter 8 the authors refer to:

The extraordinarily contrived and regulated nature of much contemporary gambling, where by design there is repetition of temporal sequences of stimuli that give pleasure whilst eroding self-control ... The behaviours themselves are all relatively simple and readily acquired, but after conditioning consistently provide access to salient positive emotion. Where else in human endeavours, in relationships, in parenting, in work, in play, are such simple dependable responses available to access similar salient positive emotion? (p. 119).

The question is raised of whether we can speak of "harm minimisation", or what the gambling industry is tending to call "responsible gambling"? The latter may be thought to imply that the fault lies with the irresponsibility of the gambler rather than the structural features of the product itself. The authors prefer the expression "low-risk gambling". Would minimising the risk inevitably clash with efforts to enhance the attractiveness of the product? The thorough investigation carried out by the Australian Productivity Commission (1999) estimated that one-third of gambling revenue came from problem gamblers. A Canadian study mentioned by Dickerson and O'Connor found that about half of all those people found to be sitting at an EGM terminal at any one time were regular gamblers with gambling problems.

Reassurance

My feeling of reassurance comes from a growing sense, much enhanced by the present work, that gambling is coming to occupy what I have long thought is its proper place near the centre of addiction studies. Dickerson and O'Connor suggest that gambling may show us, "… a potentially more transparent addictive process" (Chapter 8) because it is free of the "noise" of a psychoactive drug. As "substances" have been privileged in expert discussions about addiction, particularly drugs such as heroin and cocaine that have caused havoc in some of the most powerful countries, the field has been distorted and it has been difficult to identify the essence of addiction. In my view we have been misled into thinking that "substance dependence" or "substance misuse" is the prototype, and that "behavioural addictions" are of marginal interest. Recognising the addictive potential of gambling products – like alcohol, no "ordinary commodity" (Babor et al., 2003) – helps us reshape the field. "It is not to 'substances' that we are at risk of becoming addicted, but rather to 'objects and activities' of which drugs are a special example" (Orford, 2001, p. 2). All addictions are "behavioural addictions".

The pages of recent issues of *Addiction* are testimony to the move towards acknowledging excessive or uncontrolled gambling as an addiction. An example is Dowling et al.'s (2005) review of the evidence linking electronic gaming machines (EGMs) and gambling problems. They reviewed evidence in support of the existence of that link although they drew short of agreeing with the idea that EGMs were the "crack-cocaine of gambling" in the sense that they might stand out from other forms of gambling as being more addictive. Other work recently published in the same journal includes a number of experimental studies examining evidence for the existence of gambling addiction mental schemata in the form of attention and memory biases towards gambling-related stimuli or psychophysiological reactions to gambling-related cues (e.g. Moodie and Finnigan, 2005).

Greatly reassuring is the case study presented in Chapter 7 describing the government-funded campaign undertaken in the Australian State of Victoria.

The campaign was a response to the rise in public concern about gambling harms that quickly followed the introduction of EGMs in 1992 and the first casino in 1994 (the latter housing over 1000 EGMs, with around 30,000 in the State overall). (One poll found 84% thinking that gambling represented a serious social problem.) The campaign included both public awareness raising and the provision of treatment services (which importantly were available also for concerned "others", mainly family members, even if the problem gambler was not attending). The gambling industry became positively involved, for example agreeing to the setting up of a "customer support centre" at the casino in Melbourne.

What has been happening in Australia is undoubtedly of relevance elsewhere. In Britain, for example, gambling is in a state of flux. At the time of writing there is a Gambling Bill before the Houses of Parliament. Although it has been hailed by the Government as a move to update old fashioned gambling legislation and to provide increased protection for "children and the vulnerable", its overall impact would be a liberalisation of gambling regulation on several fronts, and it is widely expected to lead to an increase in the prevalence of problem gambling. The Government is reluctant to admit to that possibility, although it has agreed to carry out regular national prevalence surveys, and the Department of Health is carrying out consultations about ways of providing treatment for problem gambling. Notable is the shift of lead Government responsibility for gambling that occurred while the Gambling Review Body (whose recommendations formed the basis of the Gambling Bill) was sitting. Throughout most of the 20th century the Home Office had taken the lead in Britain, reflecting concern about the link between gambling and crime. The lead has now been moved to the Department for Culture, Media and Sport, and Government rhetoric is all about the rights of people to enjoy gambling like any other leisure entertainment product, and the opportunities for an industry to expand and innovate with the minimum of necessary restriction (Orford, 2005).

Amongst other things the new British Gambling Bill would legalise British-based Internet gambling, remove the demand test on new gambling outlets, remove the 24-hour rule for new casino membership, allow alcohol to be served on the gaming floor of casinos, and allow advertising of gambling products. One of the most controversial proposals is the permitting of the development of large, regional casinos and the creation of a new category of super gaming machine with unlimited stakes and prizes, up to a 1000 or more of which could be situated in a regional casino. Also controversial has been the proposal to allow the continuation of Britain's unique position as a jurisdiction that permits children to play low-stake/low-prize gaming machines (the so-called "amusements with prizes") situated in "family entertainment centres" at the seaside and elsewhere.

What is proposed for Britain fills me with dismay, as does the picture painted by Dickerson and O'Connor of escalating technical advance in the design of gambling machines and the evidence they present of the widespread experience of diminished control over gambling. But at the same time I am stimulated by their struggle to understand the phenomenon of reduced control without falling back on conventional ways of thinking about addiction and dependence. I am greatly reassured that the problem of excessive gambling is being dragged by them and others out of the wings and towards the centre stage. It is no accident that this lead should be coming from Australia where liberalisation in several States has made gambling as widely accessible as almost anywhere in the world and where there is now greater public awareness of the dangers than in most other countries.

Jim Orford
Alcohol, Drugs and Addiction Research Group
School of Psychology, The University of Birmingham
Edgbaston, Birmingham, UK

References

American Psychiatric Association (1994). *Diagnostic and Statistical Manual of Mental Disorders* (4th edn.). Washington, DC: American Psychiatric Association.

Australian Productivity Commission (APC) (1999). *Australia's gambling industries.* Report No. 10, Canberra: Ausinfo.

Babor, T., Caetano, R., Casswell, S. et al (2003) Alcohol: No Ordinary Commodity. Oxford, Oxford University Press.

Clapson, M. (1992). *A Bit of a Flutter.* Manchester: Manchester University Press.

Cooper, M.L., Frone, M.R., Russell, M. & Mudar, P. (1995). Drinking to regulate positive and negative emotions: a motivational model of alcohol use. *Journal of Personality and Social Psychology*, 69, 990–1005.

Dickerson, M. & Baron, E. (2000). Contemporary issues and future directions for research into pathological gambling. *Addiction*, 95(8), 1145–1159.

Dittmar, H. (2004). Understanding and diagnosing compulsive buying. In Coombs, R. (Ed.), *Addictive Disorders: A Practical Handbook*. New York: Wiley.

Dowling, N., Smith, D. & Thomas, T. (2005). Electronic gaming machines: are they the "crack-cocaine" of gambling? *Addiction*, 100(1), 33–45.

Griffiths, M. (1995). *Adolescent Gambling.* London: Routledge.

Hsu, L.K.G. (1990). Experimental aspects of bulimia nervosa. *Behavior Modification*, 14, 50–65.

Langer, E.J. & Roth, J. (1975). Heads I win, tails it's chance: the illusion of control as a function of the sequence of outcomes in a purely chance task. *Journal of Personality and Social Psychology*, 32, 951–955.

Lesieur, H.R. & Rosenthal, R.J. (1991). Pathological gambling: a review of the literature (prepared for the American Psychiatric Association Task Force on DSM-IV
committee on disorders of impulse control). *Journal of Gambling Studies*, 7, 5–39.

Moodie, C. & Finnigan, F. (2005). A comparison of the autonomic arousal of frequent,
infrequent and non-gamblers while playing fruit machines. *Addiction*, 100, 51–59.

Orford, J. (2001). *Excessive Appetites: A Psychological View of Addictions* (2nd edn.).
Chichester: Wiley.

Orford, J. (2005). Disabling the public interest: gambling strategies and policies for
Britain. *Addiction*, 100, 1219–1225.

Parke, J. & Griffiths, M. (2004). Gambling addiction and the evolution of the "near
miss". *Addiction Research and Theory*, 12, 407–411.

List of Tables

List of Figures

1

The Research Context

Contemporary Gambling Worldwide

Over the last three decades gambling has undergone a "profound transformation", as Reith (2003) puts it, in some of the largest markets in the world: "From being regarded as an economically marginal, politically corrupt, and morally dubious activity, it has, at the start of the twenty-first century, become a global player in the economies of North America, Europe, and Australasia." (p. 9). In jurisdictions where there has been expansion of the availability of gambling there is still an ongoing debate about whether there are net benefits to the community once the economic value of the revenue and jobs created are balanced against the social costs. The latter have mainly been expressed in terms of the incidence of problem or pathological gamblers: those individuals whose involvement in gambling has resulted in a wide range of harmful impacts impinging on themselves and those around them.

One outcome of this "transformation" has been the rapid expansion of gambling research notably in the area of problem gambling. Governments and the gambling industry have often found it a political necessity to evaluate the social impacts of legalising new or additional gambling products, whether gaming machines, casinos or lotteries. Funds have flowed to research in this process and also to support the development of policy to ameliorate the harmful impacts: policy comprising a range of strategies such as community awareness campaigns, harm minimisation and services for client problem gamblers and their families. In addition two significant national reviews of the gambling industry and its related economic and social impacts, one in the USA by the National Gambling Impact Study Commission (NGISC, 1999) and in Australia by the Productivity Commission (1999), supported by many other national studies of problem gambling, have provided a framework and direction that has already energised research activities worldwide.

1

In the broader context of the addictive behaviours there is a slowly evolving contribution of gambling research to addiction theory (Dickerson, 2003). In this context Orford (2001) was concerned that research into problem gambling did not occupy a more central position. Such research in his view had the potential to offer *"the greatest challenge to conventional wisdom on the subject, and arguably the greatest opportunity for development of a comprehensive understanding of addiction"* (p. 3) but was typically perceived at the periphery of the current understanding of addictive behaviour. This monograph might be perceived as an attempt to move gambling to a more central position. It is about one limited aspect of the rapidly developing research into gambling, limited but central to psychological conceptualisations of the addictive behaviours, and therefore with the potential to contribute to the theoretical foundations of addiction. The research focus is the ability of individuals to maintain their self-control over their level of involvement in gambling: the objective to develop an understanding of the psychological processes that erode or maintain self-control of gambling.

Historical Themes

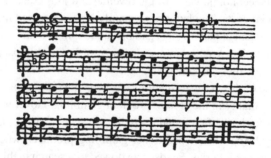

"A Lottery is a Taxation,
Upon all the Fools in Creation;
And heav'n be prais'd,
It is easily rais'd,
Credulity's always in Fashion:
For, Folly's a Fund,
Will never lose Ground,
While Fools are so rife in the nation."
(A song from ***The Lottery***, a farce by H. Fielding 1732)

Of all the contemporary forms of legalised gambling the lottery remains closest to the ancient historical origins of gambling. The lottery was one aspect of sortition, the casting or drawing of lots, a practice found in many cultures probably preceding written historical references to gambling. Ewen (1932) notes *"the simplicity with which, by means of sticks of varying length, or stones of different colour, the spoil of the chase or the booty of war could be distributed in an amicable way, or an onerous duty allotted without possibility of offensive discrimination, must have appealed to mankind when first the rights of individuals began to be recognised by the primeval community."* (p. 19)

The drawing of lots was particularly useful in the distribution of property that could not be equally divided amongst the parties involved whether it was Christ's clothes, booty from war, gifts of unequal size or government owned buildings in Tasmania. Its utility in these situations and its apparent fairness were key aspects of why the lottery became the foundation of most contemporary forms of chance-determined commercial gambling products.

The first detailed descriptions of lotteries designed to raise money for the organisers are to be found in the archives of medieval cities such as Bruges and Ghent in the Low Countries in Europe: from 1465 to 1474 thirteen lotteries were promoted in Bruges with the Duke of Burgundy taking a third of the net profit with the residue to the public purse to fund fortifications (Ewen, 1932): The forerunner of the contemporary partnership of operator and government? Certainly the language has a familiar sense of "spin". At the same time that the Portuguese were following the dictates of public relations and renaming Cape of Storms the Cape of Good Hope (Bryson, 2004), these early lotteries were described as "adventures". Regal patrons of lotteries added additional inducements. In 1569 Queen Elizabeth's "Lotterie Generall" the public announcement read:

"The Queenes Majestie, of her power royall. Giveth libertie to all manner of persons that will adventure any money in this Lotterie to resort to places underwritten ... the Citie of London ... York, Norwich, Exceter, Lincolne ... and there to remain also seven whole days, without any molestation or arrest of them for any manner of offence, saving treason, murder, pyracie or any other felonie..." (*cited by Ewen, 1932, p. 37*)

Throughout the 15th and 16th centuries lotteries were recorded throughout the German states, Italy and France. In the New World development in Virginia was aided by "adventures" organised between 1612 and 1621 but it was not until the next century that lotteries occurred regularly in Philadelphia and both Harvard and Yale in separate adventures raised and won monies for their university building funds.

The winning of millions of dollars is such a contemporary theme in the popularity of lotteries that it is somewhat surprising to find the first time such sums were advertised was 1694 in England, "The Million Lottery", authorised by Act of Parliament and interestingly paid out to winners in the form of annuities over 16 years. The long series of English State lotteries came to an end in 1826 but the first record of state prohibition occurred in Belgium in 1526 before the lottery had even crossed the Channel to England. State ambivalence toward gambling has continued throughout the world with the attraction of the possible revenues and the competing concerns from moral and religious arguments.

In the decade following the ban on lotteries in England George Adams was born, son of a farm labourer in the parish of Sandon just north of London, and who was to become associated with Australia's best known and continuing lottery, "Tatts", such a successful venture it led to the coining of an addition to the language, "to take a ticket on Tatts", to take a chance. The 16-year-old youth who landed with his parents on Circular Quay in Sydney on 28th May 1842 rapidly grew to a broad, strong man with flaming red hair and beard, taciturn yet with a ready laugh and ease in making friends. Early work at a variety of jobs followed by a period in the goldfields in Queensland led to part-ownership of a sheep station and the purchase of the Steam Packet Hotel on the south coast of New South Wales (NSW). His first involvement with gambling was when he became publican of the well-known Tattersall's Hotel in Sydney. This was the home of a sporting club set up according to the standards and rules of Tattersall's in London. In the presence of the new owner the first public Sweep, based on the 1881 running of the Sydney Cup horse race, was drawn in the main parlour of the hotel.

In a state where lotteries were banned it was inevitable that as the venture became popular, despite its reputation for integrity and fairness, the government moved to ban the sweeps in 1891. Moving to Queensland attracted similar public pressure for government to ban the sweep, but permanent stability and eventual fame came with wonderful irony in the form of the collapse of the largest bank in another state, Tasmania. With three other banks having gone into liquidation, the Bank of Van Diemen's Land was unable to withstand the run on withdrawals. It was not bankrupt, as it held a great many freehold properties, but it had to close its doors for business for lack of liquid assets and cash. Panic gripped the community and the whole economic structure of the state was threatened. After much lobbying, George Adams was invited to organise a lottery with the bank's property as the prizes (e.g. "13th Prize, Bank Premises, Devonport"). In return the Tasmanian Parliament passed a bill legalising Tattersall's sweep, and from this secure base grew what is now the largest privately owned business conglomerate in Australia.

Throughout the world today, wherever they are legalised, lotteries are the most popular form of gambling. Despite being popular it is significant that this particular form of gambling is least likely to be associated with participants' reports of impaired control over expenditure, or to result in harmful impacts, so much so that recent research has questioned whether consumption of the hypothetically most addictive form, instant or "scratch" lotteries, should be included within the mental disorder frame of reference of pathological gambling (De Fuentes-Merillas et al., 2003).

In contrast it is the relative "latecomer" to the gambling scene, the slot or fruit machine (called "poker machine" in Australia), that, wherever it has been legally and readily available, has been found to be both popular and associated with increasing community awareness of the significant harm experienced by some players and their families. Slot machines did not appear until the late 19th century in the USA, where Charles Fey transformed existing nickel in the slot machines by inventing the delayed, sequential stopping of the three reels of symbols, thereby providing what has been assumed to be the crucial element of suspense (Haw, 2000). Fey's "Liberty Bell", produced in 1899, was the forerunner of contemporary machines and found their way into casinos worldwide, notably in Nevada and also in the registered clubs in NSW, thereby adding to the existing lotteries and popular horse race meetings such as the Melbourne Cup first run in 1861 (won by "Archer", 170 pounds sterling and a gold watch), which brings Australia to a halt, with millions of dollars riding on the result (O'Hara, 1988).

Quite why Australia as a nation developed the highest participation rates in such a range of gambling activities has been the focus of scholarly debate and contemporary soul searching (Charlton, 1987; O'Hara, 1988, 1997; Costello & Millar, 2000). It is beyond the scope of this text but a personal story by the historian Ken Inglis (1985) illustrates the complex interaction of different religious beliefs and scientific progress. He relates how, brought up in a protestant family, he was "protected" from the temptations associated with betting on the Melbourne Cup by family outings, travelling deep into the bush beyond the city, arranged on the race day (a public holiday) to ensure that he and other children of like-minded parents were healthily engaged in running and sack races and the like. Catholic families enjoyed the embrace of a church more accepting of gambling and went to the racecourse. He vividly recalled the year when all this parental concern was undermined; vigorous panting youth was ordered to a silent halt while one parent attached a large wooden-cased radio to a car battery and tuned into the Cup commentary.

The clearest illustration of the outcome of a myriad of such minor struggles for and against gambling, some based on religious beliefs some on purely

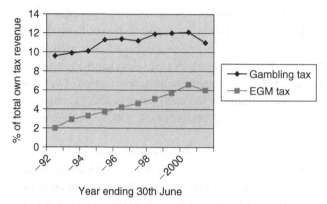

Figure 1.1. Trends in gambling tax dependency, all states and territories in Australia (adapted from Figure 3, Banks, 2003).

commercial grounds, is revealed in Figure 1.1, which shows the current dependency of Australian states and territories on the taxation revenue derived from gambling.

This drawing of the historical themes of different forms of gambling toward the present situation in Australia is driven neither by chauvinism nor a myopic worldview. It is important that any attempts to understand the processes whereby we come to both enjoy and harm ourselves from the consumption of what is described today as an "entertainment product", take account of the fact that gambling has probably been part of the human behavioural repertoire since we first understood the nature of chance.

However the focus on the Australian context is explained and justified in the following sections of this chapter, and comprises two broad themes:

1. The ready availability of the full range of contemporary gambling products within Australia permits some important causal themes to emerge that are obscured elsewhere in the world.
2. Empirical gambling data, whether describing the prevalence of harmful impacts or about player behaviours, emotions and beliefs, can only be evaluated if the community and venue context is known.

As the main empirical and conceptual thrust of this text is the bringing together of recent results that have a bearing on one, possibly key factor that causes the harmful impacts of gambling, impaired self-control, it is essential that the reader is aware of the context in which the data was collected. Only then can the conclusions drawn here, and limits to generalisation, be understood and debated. A focus on the Australian gambling context runs the risk that the research presented and discussed becomes isolated from the main body of the literature. However there is evidence in the literature that the failure to take the sometimes unique context of a particular jurisdiction or a particular type of gambling product into account has resulted in findings being inappropriately generalised to other settings, for example the association between the preference for certain gambling products and the occurrence of harmful impacts.

A detailed accounting of the Australian context *does* limit the extent to which the findings and conclusions drawn in this text hold internationally, but the potential benefits of the robust Australian data are:

1. Where generalisation can be justified the implications are stronger and more clearly identified, consolidating or challenging what is known, and
2. When findings only hold for specific contexts, types of gambling etc. the identification of these limits clarifies and may facilitate the development of new research questions.

Definitions of Gambling

No consensus appears to have been reached on a formal definition of gambling, although the aspects that distinguish it from risk-taking in general appear to be an exchange of wealth determined by a future event, the outcome of which is unknown at the time of the wager (Griffiths, 1995a). Dictionary definitions of gambling per se are almost misleadingly simple. The New Shorter Oxford Dictionary (Brown, 1993), for example, says that to gamble is to "*play games of chance for money; ... (to) risk money, fortune, success, etc., on the outcome of an event*" (p. 1057). This definition does not indicate that different forms of gambling vary greatly with regard to the probabilities governing outcomes. Most gambling in industrialised countries, such as Australia, is now structured in a manner such that a gambler can expect to lose should they persist in gambling (Walker, 1992b). This has been deemed a gambling paradox, that people should so willingly gamble when the odds are against them (Wagenaar, 1988), and most theories of "problem gambling" are attempting to explain the vigorous persistence, in the face of mounting losses, of a minority of regular gamblers.

Forms of gambling vary as to the degree of skill involved. In contrast to gambles that have minimal skill, if any (e.g. electronic gaming machines (EGMs) and roulette), are games of skill in which strict adherence to probability, coupled with experience and an aptitude for the game, can provide an advantage over an opponent (e.g. bridge, poker, blackjack – Walker, 1992b).

Somewhere on the skill continuum between the two extremes outlined above are gambling events which cannot be influenced by the gambler but involve some degree of skill. For example, horse/dog racing and sports gambling involve some skill and, notwithstanding the role of chance, will reward the more knowledgeable and skilful gambler at the expense of other gamblers (Walker, 1992b).

Legalised Forms of Gambling and their Consumption

It is neither possible to do justice to the range of gambling and gaming products that have been legalised throughout the world nor to keep pace with the development of new ones. In the present psychological research context it is helpful to classify the range of different forms into continuous and other (Dickerson, 1991): the former enabling the individual gambler to repeatedly stake, purchase a game, "observe" the outcome and repeat the process, for hours at a time. Included in this category are EGMs, off-course betting, and casino gaming, all of which have cycles of stake, play and determination ranging from 5 seconds in EGMs to several minutes for horse racing. "Other" forms are epitomised by a longer fixed period of time between the results such as the lottery drawn weekly or daily.

This distinction is at present a key factor in understanding the development of a player's impaired control over their gambling but newly developed forms of gambling product may erode the distinction. One currently available form of lottery, the instant or scratch format, where the player may purchase a quantity and "use" them one after the other in an apparent replication of a session of continuous gambling (Griffiths, 1990), appears to bridge the "gap" between lotteries and EGMs. Recent prevalence studies from the Netherlands challenge this hypothesis showing such low levels of harmful impacts for excessive users of this gambling product that the authors questioned the validity of its inclusion within the Diagnostic and Statistical Manual for Mental Disorders – 4th edn. (DSM-IV) pathological gambling frame of reference (De Fuentes-Merillas et al., 2003).

The second distinction that is essential to an understanding of the research into the psychological processes that contribute to the erosion of a gambler's self-control was made by the Productivity Commission (1999): the division of the gaming machine market into three segments:

"high-intensity machines – where spending per game and the speed of play is high relative to all other gaming machines – includes Australian gaming machines, US slot machines and video lottery terminals;

amusement with prizes machines – where spending and the speed of play is relatively slower – these include UK amusement with prizes...

Japanese pinball style pachinko and other machines (such as the UK crane grab) – where the stakes and speed of play are the lowest and the prizes are toys and biscuits, cigarettes...." (p. 2.11)

Table 1.1. *A comparison of gaming machine density for selected jurisdictions in Canada and Australia*

Jurisdiction	Total EGMs	EGMs/adult
New South Wales (Australia)	102,000	1:40
Victoria (Australia)	32,500	1:90
Nova Scotia	3,959	1:180
Newfoundland	2,539	1:162
New Brunswick	2,795	1:206
Quebec	20,421	1:275
Alberta	10,352	1:208
British Columbia	2,175	1:1409

Adapted from Azmier, 2001.

The majority of the high-intensity EGMs are in US casinos (64.4%), but there are 20% in Australia, half of them within the one state, NSW, where the research reported in the following chapters was conducted.

Consumption of Gambling

The consumption of gambling varies greatly worldwide reflecting the availability of the different gambling products. In the USA the annual per capita expenditure was estimated at $238 in 1997 with 60% of the population gambling during 1998 (NGISC, 1999). In the UK about 70% of the population participate in gambling in any one year with the annual per capita expenditure of 155BP (in $ about $226) (Sproston et al., 2000). In Australia over 80% of the population participate in gambling in any one year (Productivity Commission, 1999) and by 2000–2001 the annual per capita expenditure had grown to A$1000 (double the expenditure in the USA and UK), over half of which was spent on EGM play (Banks, 2003). Similarly over half of the revenue arises from EGMs whether in clubs, hotels or casinos that is over 5% of own-tax revenues (excluding federally allocated income).

It is the availability of EGMs in venues associated with the day-to-day work and leisure routines of most Australians (with the exception of Western Australia (WA)) combined with a high machine density per adult member of the population (e.g. in NSW 1 per 40) that is so very different from almost every other jurisdiction worldwide. In Canada some provinces approach similar levels and this is summarised in Table 1.1. In Nova Scotia for example the density of EGMs (video lottery terminals) is about 1 per 180 adults, once again available in hotels/bars as well as casinos (Schrans & Schellinck, 2004).

In NSW just over 10% of the population play EGMs once per week or more often (Dickerson et al., 1998) (are "regular" players, Productivity Commission, 1999). Although the proportion of such regular players in Nova Scotia is much lower (2.4%, Schrans & Shellinck, 2004) the similarities in the type of EGMs and their "convenience" availability goes some way to explaining the similarity of the research findings in the two jurisdictions and this important contextual theme is further discussed later in this chapter.

Definitions: Excessive, Problem and Pathological Gambling

"I do not know if there is any other passion which allows less of repose and which one has so much difficulty in reducing ... the passion of gambling gives no time for breathing ... it is a persecutor, furious and indefatigable. The more one plays the more one wishes to play. With difficulty one resolves to leave off a little to satisfy the needs of nature ... it seems that gambling had acquired the rights to occupy all his thoughts." (Jean Barbeyrac, 1737; cited in Orford, 2001)

Excessive Gambling

Excessive gambling (Orford, 2001) indicates a level of involvement and appetite for gambling that clashes with restraints (e.g. monetary, time, requirements of relationships, work obligations, values of the gambler or others) on an individual's gambling. It could be argued that the word "excessive" has moral overtones, that what is considered excessive may be vaguely defined and highly subjective (Walker, 1992b). However, an appealing aspect of the term "excessive gambling" is that it can apply to the situation where no problems are as yet in evidence, but nevertheless a potential for harm exists. Perhaps the gambling field needs an array of terms analogous to the framework adopted by the World Health Organisation (1982) for alcohol and other drug problems. In addition to the recognition of dependence, there are the terms "unsanctioned use" (quite simply, some people disapprove of the behaviour), "hazardous use" (there exists the potential for harm), "dysfunctional use" (there is disruption to relationships and performance) and "harmful use" (direct harm can be measured).

To a large extent, definitions of excessive gambling are often more implicit in a theoretical stance than made explicit in the difficult task of an all-encompassing definition (Walker, 1992b). Nevertheless, attempts at definition are made to satisfy clinical, research and policy requirements.

Problem Gambling

The terms "problem gambling" have commonly been used to indicate a level less severe than "pathological" and this is formalised in the labelling of cut-off points in measures such as the South Oaks Gambling Screen (SOGS) (Lesieur & Blume, 1987). In some jurisdictions problem gambling has been used not only to refer to all psychological and social issues associated with gambling in part to avoid the medicalisation of the debate but also to ensure that policy was comprehensive and strategies adopted went far beyond the delivery of services to individuals in need.

More recently, the Australian Institute for Gambling Research has defined "problem gambling" as *"the situation where a person's gambling activity gives rise to harm to the individual player, and/or to his or her family, and may extend into the community"* (Dickerson, et al., 1997; p. 106). Definitions such as this imply that gambling involvement rests on a continuum, from occasional non-problematic levels, through to extreme over-involvement with attendant problems. Harm can range from the relatively minor and transient to a host of chronic problems that may be accompanied by a sense of impaired self-control (Dickerson, 1991). The classification of the harms into interpersonal, intrapersonal, vocational/educational, economic and legal has been used as the basis for surveys of the general population (e.g. Dickerson et al., 1996a, b, 1998).

In Australia, where most states and territories have not preferred the mental disorder model as the basis for their policy development, the above definition in some senses reflected current usage and deliberately avoided any theoretical causal assumptions. This was in a community setting where the acceptance of legalised gambling was generally high, with up to 90% of the population participating in gambling in any 12-month period. The definition maintained the focus on the harmful impacts of gambling, a concern shared by all stakeholders, the government, the industry and the community. In a multicultural community it also emphasised that the problems arising from gambling could be strongly determined by social and cultural context. The definition provides a contrast with the mental disorder model, as it is based on observable outcomes "outside" the individual, an approach to defining addiction vehemently criticised (Aasved, 2003).

Pathological Gambling

Whilst the terms "problem gambling" and "excessive gambling" imply a point of departure from non-problematic/excessive gambling, these definitions allow

Table 1.2 *Diagnostic criteria for pathological gambling (DSM-IV, APA, 1994)*

A: Persistent and recurrent maladaptive gambling behaviour as indicated by five (or more) of the following:
  1. Is preoccupied with gambling (e.g. preoccupied with reliving past gambling experiences, handicapping* or planning the next venture, or thinking of ways to get money with which to gamble);
  2. Needs to gamble with increasing amounts of money in order to achieve the desired excitement;
  3. Has repeated unsuccessful efforts to control, cut back, or stop gambling;
  4. Is restless or irritable when attempting to cut down or stop gambling;
  5. Gambles as a way of escaping from problems or of relieving a dysphoric mood (e.g. feelings of helplessness, guilt, anxiety, depression);
  6. After losing money gambling, often returns another day to get even ("chasing" one's losses);
  7. Lies to family members, therapists, or others to conceal the extent of involvement with gambling;
  8. Has committed illegal acts such as forgery, fraud, theft, or embezzlement to finance gambling;
  9. Has jeopardised or lost a significant relationship, job, or educational career opportunity because of gambling;
  10. Relies on others to provide money to relieve a desperate financial situation caused by gambling.

B: The gambling behaviour is not better accounted for by a manic episode.**

* Studying the form.
** Another diagnosis within the DSM-IV.

for that point to be individually and socially referenced in each case, rather than fixed by an arbitrary number of diagnostic criteria. Extreme cases of problem gambling often attract the label "pathological gambling" (APA, 1994) or, less frequently now, "compulsive gambling". A dichotomy of pathological or compulsive gambling on the one hand, and social gambling on the other, mirrors the now obsolete distinction between "alcoholism" and "social drinking" (Heather & Robertson, 1989). The World Health Organisation (Edwards et al., 1977) has long eschewed the concept of "alcoholism" as a discrete entity, and instead recommended the use of the term "alcohol-related problems". However, the notion that heavier levels of drinking and drug taking are usually associated with a greater degree of dependency, accompanied by a sense of impaired control, was retained.

The most widely used psychiatric criteria for the diagnosis of "pathological gambling" are those contained in the DSM-IV (APA, 1994: see Table 1.2). They appear to be of clinical relevance, but it is debatable as to whether it is warranted, or desirable, to reach a firm diagnosis on the basis of any 5 of the 10 criteria. Given the lack of weighting on any particular criterion, no confidence can be had that such a procedure will reliably distinguish those who have significant problems from those who do not (Wakefield, 1997). Wakefield has argued that DSM-IV criteria generally are so inclusive as to fail to distinguish serious psychological dysfunction from "problems in living". Since the original examination of the diagnostic items comparing self-identified pathological gamblers and substance abusers (Lesieur & Rosenthal, 1991), research into the validity and reliability of the clinical usage of the DSM-IV diagnostic criteria of pathological gambling has yet to be published. The National Research Council Report (1999) asserted that "*the DSM-IV criteria appear to have worked well for clinicians for the past five years*" (p. 27) but provided no evidence in support.

The great advantage of psychosocial definitions, as opposed to psychiatric diagnostic criteria, is that they do not imply that the excessive gambler is mentally ill. A parallel was observed in the transition from "alcoholism" to problem drinking; Heather and Robertson (1989) stated that it brought alcohol problems back into the realm of "normal" and everyday drinking, allowing models to be built on typical processes rather than clinical or pathological worse-case scenarios. More fluid and relative definitions also allow for anyone who regularly drinks (or gambles) to, potentially, develop a problem under certain circumstances, thus removing undue emphasis on individual differences at the expense of conditioning and structural variables (Heather & Robertson, 1989). These themes anticipate much of the findings for regular gamblers in this monograph.

Measures of Excessive, Problem and Pathological Gambling

Following the seminal prevalence study by Volberg & Steadman (1988) the SOGS (Lesieur & Blume, 1987) became the standard instrument over the next decade. Comprising a heterogeneous set of questions about difficulties controlling gambling, negative feelings about gambling and emphasising the borrowing of monies to support gambling, it was validated in a clinical setting using a criterion group of diagnosed pathological gamblers (DSM-III, APA, 1980) and a comparison convenience sample. Despite setting a cut-off point for identifying those with the mental disorder, "at any time in the past" (lifetime version), it was typically used as if individuals could be placed on a continuum of levels of problem severity and the "the last 12 months" format was developed and preferred (Abbott and Volberg, 1992). Shaffer et al. (1997) in the first meta-analysis of prevalence studies aided the debate by linking the threshold of cut-offs with the criteria of relevance to policy, proposing Levels I–III with the latter representing severe problems requiring intervention or treatment.

A major concern raised about the SOGS was the base-rate issue and the resultant loss of specificity when the screen was used in general population studies for which it was not designed (Culleton, 1989; Dickerson, 1993; Walker & Dickerson, 1996). In Australia the screen was used extensively but the cut-point for pathological gambling was taken as an indication of "at risk" of significant harmful impacts from gambling and the term "problem" gambler was preferred. (As discussed at Chapter 7 in no state was funding of, or access to, free services for problem gamblers made contingent upon the diagnosis of pathological gambling and therefore government funded research was not required to provide prevalence estimates in terms of pathological gambling.) The approach used to reduce the false positive rates of the SOGS in all previous studies completed in Australia were independently reviewed by the Productivity Commission (1999), and incorporated into the Commission's own first national survey using the SOGS (e.g. the "Dickerson method").

The other main source of measures has been the DSM-IV diagnostic items themselves, but the scales, whether designed for use with children (Fisher, 1992) or for the national survey in the USA (NORC, 1999), have been weakened by the assumption that basic psychometric criteria of reliability and validity need not be satisfied. There have been no psychometrically satisfactory studies confirming that the "cases" identified by the scales were indeed pathological gambling, nor was the accuracy of the cut-off point evaluated: it assumed to be same as in the diagnostic criteria despite that fact that this was decided not by the American Psychiatric Association expert committee on gambling but by the central organising body determining the final form of the DSM-IV. When used concurrently with the SOGS scales derived from the DSM-IV, the scales have tended to yield slightly lower prevalence estimates (e.g. Sproston et al., 2001).

A more promising measure has been the recent development of the Canadian Problem Gambling Index (CPGI) (Ferris & Wynne, 2001). This is a 30-item scale assessing participation in gambling, harmful impacts and demographics, nine of which are scored to give a Problem Gambling Severity Index (PGSI). Problem gambling is again conceptualised as a continuum from "Non-problem gambler", through "At risk", to "Moderate problem" to "Severe problem" (latest category labels from Wiebe et al., 2001). Concurrent validation with the SOGS was used in the original development (Ferris & Wynne, 2001) to enable the scores on the severity index to be matched with the commonly used categories on the established measure.

One published study has endeavoured to break out of the psychological/psychiatric frame of reference (Ben-Tovim et al., 2001). The second in a sequence that set out to first define (Dickerson et al., 1997) and then measure problem gambling, the most difficult task was the definition and measurement of "harm". An expert judgment method was adopted. Items for the scale, called the Victorian Gambling Screen (VGS), were derived from the literature and from focus group studies. The project progressed through several pilot stages to a main validation study. The latter resulted in a scale of 21 items that gave a three-factor structure comprising harm to the individual, to the partner, and the respondent's enjoyment of gambling. Based on the Receiver Operator Characteristic (ROC) technique that plots test sensitivity against specificity, the results showed that the harm-to-self scale showed a clear and sudden transition associated with only modest misclassification rates for problem gamblers and non-problem gamblers.

Similarities between the CPGI and the then emerging VGS, both placed far greater emphasis than previous measures on the harmful impacts of gambling and the environmental events that may contribute to problem gambling (Productivity Commission, 1999). An independent evaluation of the VGS and other population screens preferred the new CPGI (GRP, 2004).

Prevalence of Problem Gambling

The first published meta-analysis of prevalence studies carried out in the US and Canada (Shaffer et al., 1997) identified 152 studies, 120 of which met the inclusion criteria. Apart from the prevalence rates themselves which more recent national studies have superceded, the report proposed the use of three levels of severity of problems in order to assist comparisons across methods and jurisdictions and also emphasised the necessary linkage of prevalence methodology and policy objectives; both contributed to advance this aspect of gambling research.

The lack of an established international prevalence methodology for assessing problem gambling has made comparisons between jurisdictions difficult. In the US the first national survey since 1976 (Kallick et al., 1976) preferred an entirely new measure based on the DSM-IV (APA, 1994) diagnostic items for pathological gambling (NORC, 1999) and estimated that between 0.6% and 0.9% of the population were pathological gamblers and a further 0.7–2.0 were problem gamblers. The sensitivity and specificity of this new screen were not adequately demonstrated and cut-off points were not statistically validated. In Australia 2.1% scored 5 or more on the SOGS, the cut-point for pathological gambling but the authors, the Productivity Commission (1999), in order to reduce the predicted false positives estimated that only half were experiencing severe problems (Level III, Shaffer et al., 1997). In the UK both the SOGS and the DSM-IV screens were used concurrently in the first national survey (Sproston et al., 2001). Prevalence rates of gamblers experiencing problems in the last year were reported for each scale of 0.82% and 0.62% respectively.

Other national studies using the SOGS cut-point of 5 or more have published prevalence estimates: 0.6% in Sweden (Ronneberg et al., 1999), in New Zealand 0.3–0.7% Level III and 0.6–1.1% Level II (Department of Internal Affairs, 2001), in Canada using the CPGI, 0.9% Level III and 2.4% Level II (Ferris & Wynne, 2001). Accurate international comparisons await the resolution or methodological and even sampling issues, for example Schellinck & Schrans (2003) estimated that the usual method of population sampling by telephone of one person per household, compared with interviewing randomly selected *households* (all adults) may over-estimate problem gambling prevalence by 23%.

Despite the difficulties in making comparisons it has been concluded, supported by the per capita expenditure data, that levels of problem gambling are higher in Australia than most jurisdictions (Productivity Commission, 1999).

Repeated measures of prevalence in the same jurisdiction were pioneered by Volberg (e.g. In New York, 1996) but are exceedingly demanding given the low proportion of "cases" and the often rapidly changing availability of gambling products, of the exact characteristics of the products and therefore in the level of involvement in gambling reported by the community. Repeated prevalence measures if they include an analysis of such changes and perhaps a cost-benefit analysis of the industry and related social costs may provide a basis for policy (e.g. Dickerson et al., 1998). Such attempts at costing have been positively evaluated (NRC, 1999), but the assumptions of the economic model underpinning such attempts have been challenged (Productivity Commission, 1999). One of the most informative prevalence studies included a follow-up of "cases" identified in the previous survey some 7 years earlier; both were carried out by Max Abbott, Rachel Volberg and colleagues in New Zealand (Department of Internal Affairs, 2001).

Risk Factors: Emerging Causal Themes

The wealth of prevalence studies has enabled a framework to be developed that provides some insight into the origins of problem gambling. Risk factors are necessarily a function of a particular gambling context and may not necessarily be generalised to another jurisdiction unless the situation is similar. This is clarified below by first presenting survey and clinical data (Dickerson et al.,

1997; Productivity Commission, 1999) indicating that risk factors in Australia include:

(i) increased accessibility to legalised gambling;

(ii) "continuous" forms of gambling such as EGMs, horse/dog betting and casino gaming (as opposed to other forms such as lotto, pools and bingo that do not permit continuous cycles of stake, play and determination);

(iii) being less than 25 years of age doubles the risk (with young males at greatest risk);

(iv) living in urban rather than in rural areas;

(v) for women who gamble regularly, a preference for EGMs;

(vi) earning slightly less than an average income;

(vii) being separated, divorced, unemployed and living in single-person dwellings (direction of causality unknown);

(viii) being socially and economically disadvantaged and having ready access to gambling. There is evidence in Australia that people of some non-English speaking backgrounds may be over-represented in problem gambling (VCGA, 2000), and evidence from elsewhere that Indigenous people are at greater risk (Volberg & Abbott, 1997).

Access and Continuous Forms

The first two listed are by far the most significant factors and require clarification and expansion. Prior to 1992 EGMs were legalised only in one state and one territory in Australia and clinical experience at the time provided examples of clients who satisfied the diagnostic criteria of pathological gambling in one state, but on moving to take up employment in another, were "cured". Access to legalised gambling is an obvious risk factor but *ease* of access can also be very significant. At the moment betting by phone and Internet gambling from home remain a tiny proportion of the gambling market. The majority of gambling takes place in licensed, highly regulated venues. Some venues are limited to one or two per state in the form of casinos, some are better considered in terms of *"convenience access"* such as the EGM rooms in hotels, bars and social clubs throughout all states and territories except WA where EGMs are available only within the casino.

If the very small EGM market in Tasmania (i.e. in 1999) is excluded it is notable that the prevalence rate (SOGS score 5) in WA was lower than all others by a factor of two and almost four times smaller than for the state with the greatest number of EGMs, NSW (0.7% versus 2.55% respectively) (Productivity

Commission, 1999). As the accessibility to all other types of gambling product are very similar across jurisdictions it is reasonable to argue that it is not just availability but convenience access that is an especially powerful risk factor. Where EGMs are in venues that are on the daily routes of people going to and from work (open 24 hours) and part of the facilities of leisure and entertainment centres within a short drive or walk from home then regular EGM sessions (weekly and more often) are reported by 10% of the general population (Dickerson et al., 1998). In another state, Victoria, which has the second largest number of EGMs and similar convenience access, recent prevalence research found that three-quarters of the prevalence of 2.45% could be attributed to playing EGMs (ACIL, 2001, cited in Banks, 2003).

It may prove necessary in future research to operationalise convenience access in ways similar to alcohol research, such as geographical dispersion of venues (Stockwell & Gruenewald, 2001). When EGMs were first introduced to Victoria the Victorian Casino and Gaming Authority developed a unique computer-based machine density map by region of the state. Recent survey data from the same state found that 32.5% of people travelled less than 3 km to play EGMs and a further 25% less than 5 km (GRP, 2004). Recent research has approached the problem from the perspective of geographical dispersion of social disadvantage and access to gambling in casinos (Welte et al., 2004).

At present the most useful indicator of ease of access is the assumed outcome, regular gambling, and this is a strong indicator of risk of the harmful impacts that can arise from gambling. Regular gambling has typically been combined with the second risk factor, continuous forms versus other, and used as a basis for the design of prevalence studies in Australia (e.g. Dickerson & Baron, 1994a, b; Dickerson et al. 1996a, b, 1998; Productivity Commission, 1999). In Table 1.3 it must be noted that "Lottery only" means that the respondent did not consume continuous forms on a *regular* basis but most did so less frequently than weekly. In contrast those who regularly used continuous forms would also typically purchase some type of lottery product regularly as well.

Comparisons of level of involvement, for example, frequency of gambling *within* one particular form of continuous gambling such as EGM play illustrate the very significant increase in risk associated with regularity of gambling. Taking a SOGS score of 5 or more as the "definition" of a problem gambler, this gives the following probabilities for any individual being a problem gambler:

- for the general adult population in Australia, $p = 0.02$;
- for all EGM players, $p = 0.047$;
- for regular EGM players, $p = 0.226$ (Productivity Commission, 1999).

Table 1.3 *Regular players, lottery versus those who prefer betting and gaming (continuous forms)*

| Player type | N | Reports of negative impact by type of impact* | | | | |
		Personal %	Family %	Financial %	Vocation %	Legal %
Lottery only	(140)	63	7	14	3	3
Betting & EGM regulars	(159)	84	44	45	10	10

*%s total more than 100/row as respondents could check more than one type of impact. (Adapted from Dickerson et al., 1996.)

A study in Nova Scotia, another jurisdiction with convenience access to EGMs, was able to take this one step further illustrating how the probability of any one player actually sitting playing an EGM (video lottery terminal) being a regular *and* a problem gambler was about $p = 0.5$, varying slightly according to the day of the week and the hour of the day (Schellinck & Schrans, 1998). This was based on the fact that regular players not only entered the venue more frequently than other players but also when problematic levels were reached, stayed for almost twice as long per session of play.

The study of risk levels within other continuous forms of gambling such as off-course betting and casino table games show very similar patterns of increased risk for regular gamblers. However, because a much smaller proportion of the population regularly consume these, compared with EGM play their contribution to prevalence levels is correspondingly smaller. This is not to say that EGM play is more "addictive", the proportion at risk is very similar across the regular player base of all continuous forms of gambling (e.g. Productivity Commission, 1999; see also discussion in Chapter 6) and for example the preponderance of EGM excessive players amongst the new clients of problem gambling services (see Chapter 7) is primarily a function of the popularity of EGM play and its significantly larger regular player base than for any other continuous form.

The risk factors of access/regular consumption and continuous form of gambling product make sense of both the higher expenditure per capita and the higher prevalence rates found in Australia compared with other jurisdictions worldwide. In other jurisdictions it is rare for continuous forms to have convenience access and support regular gambling sessions (i.e. weekly and more frequent consumption). Random population prevalence surveys will therefore tend to recruit only a small number of such regular players and the association with increased risk in the context of much lower overall prevalence rates will be very much more difficult to detect. In addition it is possible that where the "full" range of gambling products are easily accessible then it is rare for an individual who regularly gambles on lotteries only to gamble excessively. (In over 20 years of clinical experience of counselling, supervising and evaluating problem gambling services the authors have recorded only one such individual.) In other jurisdictions this may be more common in the absence of access or convenience access to continuous forms. Given the much lower prevalence levels in jurisdictions where lottery products are the only form with convenience access it can be argued that the "development" of excessive consumption may be more difficult for lottery than continuous types of gambling product. What is clear is that generalisation of risk factors from one jurisdiction to another must not be assumed without supporting evidence.

Research Requirements

Ellen Langer (1975) in her study of the illusion of control used a sequence of ecologically valid settings, one of which was a lottery purchase, primarily because during pilot studies she had found the phenomenon difficult to demonstrate in the laboratory. The need for ecological validity was specifically evaluated for gambling by the seminal study of Anderson & Brown (1984). They provided a striking demonstration that gambling behaviour is contextually sensitive and may alter significantly depending on the ecological validity of the research design. In a "convincing" laboratory casino students and regular gamblers played blackjack for prizes; subsequently the latter were also observed actually playing blackjack (their preferred game) in their preferred local casino. In the laboratory heart rate increases ranged from 4 to 7 beats/minute, in the casino the mean rate of increase was 23.1 beats/minute and ranged as high as 58 beats per minute. Predicted relationships between stake size and personality were not supported in the laboratory but were strongly confirmed in the venue. Patterns of staking were significantly different from one setting to the other. These results together with similar contrasting results for gaming machines from ecologically valid settings (e.g. Leary & Dickerson, 1985; Moodie & Finnigan, 2005) and artificial laboratory methods (e.g. Rule et al., 1971) confirmed the sensitivity to context of gambling behaviours, emotions and cognitions.

Arguments have been made in defence of laboratory studies of gambling (Ladouceur, 1991; Walker, 1992a) but both authors have more recently preferred more ecologically valid settings and methods (e.g. Ladouceur et al., 2003; Blaszczynski et al., 2001). If laboratory methods or analogue studies have a place in model building they need to involve an opportunity to actually lose and win cash and to recruit participants who currently consume a similar gambling product. Even under these conditions results need subsequent testing in ecologically valid settings.

In this context it was argued:

"Implicit in much of the work on excessive or pathological gambling has been the assumption that impaired control arises in a similar fashion whether the person plays poker machines (i.e. EGMs), bets, plays roulette or engages in another preferred form of gambling. Given the very different stimulus and temporal characteristics of the different forms, such an assumption has poor face validity. It is further undermined by the fact that some gamblers use one form exclusively, showing impaired control of that form and that form alone." (Dickerson, 1993, p. 226)

Acknowledging the significance and heterogeneity of the person–situation interaction in gambling activities raises the possibility that by establishing the different conditions under which impaired self-control arises insight may be gained into the underlying psychological processes. For example, it may be speculated that in terms of generating similar levels of impaired control in regular off-course gamblers and EGM players, the much slower temporal sequence of the former may be "compensated" by significant emotional changes for each bet placed. Detailed comparisons between the different forms of gambling may provide a conceptual model of impaired self-control that is applicable to other addictive behaviours.

2

Research into Impaired Control of Gambling Behaviour, Definition and Measurement: Traditional Psychometric and Mathematical Psychology Approaches

Gambling as One of the Addictions

Gambling, and the harm that can arise from the expenditure of time and money on gambling, has been included amongst the addictive behaviours for several decades (Marlatt, 1979). The absence of a psychoactive agent did not give rise to any serious challenge to its inclusion amongst the addictive behaviours (although anecdotally it was associated with sceptical enquiries such as, "Can I become addicted to gardening?"). The contemporary issue has moved on to question where the boundary should be placed with regard to activities such as exercise, shopping and most recently, Internet usage (Griffiths, 1999a).

Psychological models of the addictions are unlikely to provide the basis for some clear dividing line or "addictive" category because core explanatory themes such as self-control, learning and individual differences are all conceptualised as dimensions of essentially normal human functioning. Orford (2001) gives three strong pragmatic, rather than theoretical, reasons for limiting the category of excessive or addictive behaviours to six behaviours; alcohol, eating, straight sex, tobacco, hard drugs and gambling because:

1. They are the best documented examples.
2. They involve behaviours typically enjoyed by most people without encountering problems but which as addictions cause enormous human distress and suffering.
3. The "danger of trivialising the debate about addiction if the concept is extended too far" (p. 5).

This is not to say that other apparently addictive behaviours should not be considered. In fact, any psychological account of the processes that cause a person to become addicted should also provide insight into all the combinations of types of human behaviours, situations and subjective experiences that are likely to place a person at risk of addiction.

If it can, therefore, be assumed that gambling is one of the core addictive behaviours, then what is the nature of the research task? The most obvious question is, "Why for most people is the consumption of any of a wide range of gaming and betting products a pleasurable and harm-free leisure activity but for some becomes addictive?" "Addictive" implies that the associated harmful impacts arising from gambling are deeply distressing for the individual, significantly damaging their interpersonal relations and all aspects of their lives, and even the social fabric of the community in which they live.

The "pathways model of problem and pathological gambling" (Blaszczynski & Nower, 2002) provides a helpful summary of the complexity of the research task (Figure 2.1).

The three pathways that describe the progression from gambling to problem or pathological gambling consist of the following:

- Pathway 1: A conditioning process leading to habitual levels of involvement and associated behaviours of chasing losses and losing excessively.
- Pathway 2: Interactions between the learning process (Pathway 1) and emotional and biological vulnerabilities.
- Pathway 3: Includes the same interaction as for Pathways 1 and 2, but within a specifically identified group *"distinguished by features of impulsivity and antisocial personality disorder"* (p. 494).

The authors believe that there are sub-types of problem gamblers, ranging from the essentially normal regular gambler who moves into and out of excessive levels of expenditure but with few other harmful impacts, to the other extreme of the essentially mentally disordered gambler whose symptoms satisfy the diagnostic and statistical manual of mental disorders, 4th edition (DSM-IV) criteria for pathological gambling, and who may also have personality disturbance and co-morbid disorders such as alcohol dependence. They view attempts to explain such disparate types from a single theoretical perspective as essentially a fool's errand. The pathways model classified many different theoretical approaches according to which sub-type of problem gambling it is most likely to explain. In a most convincing manner, the review demonstrated the breadth of emerging evidence regarding the origins of pathological gambling from the twin studies of Eisen et al. (1998) to research suggesting the possible inherited differences in neurotransmitter systems (Comings et al., 1996) and to work studying the altered functioning of such systems in pathological gamblers (Bergh et al., 1997). Also strongly emphasised was the evidence of associations

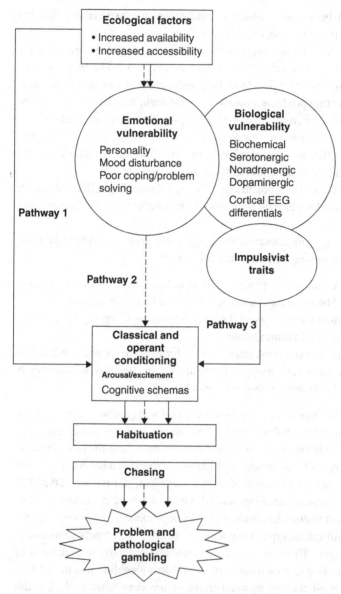

Figure 2.1. The "pathways model of problem and pathological gambling" (Blaszczynski & Nower, 2002).

between pathological gambling and other mental disorders such as mood disorders (e.g. Beaudoin & Cox, 1999) and antisocial personality disorder Blaszczynski et al. (1997). In addition, Blaszczynski & Nower (2002) explored the clinical implications of the model for the treatment and management of the different types of problem gambling.

Throughout the following presentation of empirical findings and arguments this model will be used as a way of exploring the implications and for testing generalisations: the model serves as a bridge between the more limited focus of the present research and the broad field of problem gambling.

Problem Gambling as the Dependent Variable

The origins of most of the research to be presented in the following sections of this and the next chapter are associated with the deliberate attempt to conduct research that was neither burdened nor restricted by the clinical context of treating and "explaining" pathological gambling. The goal was to tread that fine line between gaining the benefits of simplifying the research task and enabling the use of stronger research methods, and yet maintaining the relevance of the research questions and outcomes to the realities of the harmful impacts experienced by problem and pathological gamblers.

This approach was first articulated in Dickerson & Baron (2000). That article emphasised that it was the heterogeneity of the symptoms included in the diagnostic criteria for pathological gambling that was undermining the outcomes of the contemporary focus of research on the mental disorder model of gambling. Symptoms ranging from actual gambling behaviours, to lying to family members, to theft and fraud, presented the psychological researcher with a supremely difficult task: how to select a manageable group of psychological constructs that might account for the diverse harmful impacts and gambling behaviour, and how to ensure the independence of measures of predictor variables.

The question of whether it is possible to separate the harmful impacts of gambling from the gambling behaviour itself, and still be able to conduct research that is relevant to the underlying addictive process, is a complex and fraught issue. Certainly the DSM-IV criteria permit the diagnosis of pathological gambling to be made without the inclusion of harmful impacts, but based entirely upon gambling related behaviours, attitudes and thoughts (criteria 1–6 see Chapter 1). However, it is rare for individual gamblers to seek help unless they are experiencing several distressing harmful impacts. In addition, it is well established that these harmful impacts, whether debts, dysphoria or theft, are strong predictors of continued excessive gambling. In other words, as well illustrated in Orford et al. (1996) in a model of attachment to gambling, the harmful impacts feed a cycle of increasing strength of attachment and continuing harmful outcomes. The separation of these harmful impacts from the addictive behaviour, the gambling itself, may therefore be quite artificial and may risk removal of the actual addictive process from the research endeavour.

When the question is considered in the broader context of the addictive behaviours generally, the "removal" of the harmful impacts might be taken to mean that the research focus was no longer on an addiction. Thus in the DSM-IV (American Psychiatric Association (APA), 1994) and international classification of diseases (ICD)-10 (WHO, 1992) criteria for Substance Abuse and Harmful Abuse, the criteria *require* the presence of harmful impacts. However, the criteria for alcohol dependence in both classificatory systems is similar to that for gambling, as the diagnosis can be made without the requirement that there are specified harmful impacts, the harm perhaps being implicit in the drinking related behaviours, for example evidence of tolerance such that increased dosages are required, relief drinking to prevent the onset of withdrawal, a lack of discrimination in choice of drinking situations when drinking assumes an over-riding salience in the persons' life.

The question of just what is the "addictive process" does not go away, and we return to this fundamental issue throughout the text. At this stage it is sufficient to indicate awareness that the attempt to focus gambling research, and thereby possibly addiction research, on a more homogeneous dependent variable that excludes the harmful impacts of gambling may have very significant theoretical costs, despite the methodological and research benefits that accrue.

Self-control as the Dependent Variable in Problem Gambling Research

The impairment of the ability of individuals to control their expenditure of time and money spent on gambling has been described in terms of "gambling longer than intended", "spending more than planned" and "spending more than can be afforded", and surveys of player and clinical samples has shown it to be a very common experience Corless & Dickerson (1989). It has been argued that, "*It is difficult to reject the premise that the erosion of a person's ability to control their time and money expenditure on gambling is central to the psychological understanding of the origins of the harm that can arise.*" (Dickerson & Baron, 2000, p. 1149). Self-control of gambling behaviour was defined in terms of consistently staying within preferred levels of involvement that is time and money expenditure. The objective of subsequent research was conceptualised as an examination of the psychological variables that lead to the erosion and/or maintenance of self-control over gambling. It was assumed that the impairment of self-control experienced/reported by gamblers and problem gamblers differed in degree only, and that the erosion of self-control represented the core addictive process that drove the harmful impacts. It was therefore assumed that psychological research into the addictive process underlying problem gambling could validly focus on current regular gamblers using the full spectrum of research methods, rather than depending on the retrospective reports of problem gamblers entering treatment.

This emphasis on self-control is compatible with research more firmly based within the mental disorder model of pathological gambling, and with research into the addictions generally. For example, in the pathways model of pathological gambling, Blaszczynski & Nower (2002) identify impaired control, defined in terms of "repeated unsuccessful attempts to resist the urge in the context of a genuine desire to cease, as the central, diagnostic and foundational feature of pathological gambling" (p. 488). The caveat of the genuine desire to become abstinent is a significant difference from Dickerson & Baron's (2000) definition, and the authors went on to construe this impaired control as a "*disordered or diseased state that deviates from normal, healthy behaviour*" (Blaszczynski & Nower, 2002, p. 488). The authors also imply that there is a qualitative difference between the impairment of self-control reported by regular gamblers who become problem/pathological gamblers as a result of classical and operant conditioning processes (Pathway 1) and other "true" pathological gamblers whose origins are described by the other two pathways. For Blaszczynski & Nower (2002), the impaired control exhibited by the former, regular gamblers is not true impairment of self-control, but a function of the conditioning experience, inaccurate estimations of probabilities and poor decision-making.

These differences in the definition and conceptualisation of impaired self-control over gambling present potential barriers or limitations to generalising from some of the results presented below and will be re-examined later.

In the context of other addictive behaviours, the research focus on impaired self-control can be readily defended, but there are differences in emphasis placed on the construct. For example, compared with pathological gambling, the diagnosis of alcohol dependence includes, rather than emphasises, subjective control: the alcohol dependence syndrome (ADS) specified the subjective awareness of a compulsion to drink as one of seven dimensions and the diagnostic criteria for the DSM-IV (APA, 1994) and the ICD-10 (WHO, 1992) each include two items (of a total of seven and six, respectively) that refer specifically to aspects of impaired control over consumption. Nonetheless, in both systems the diagnosis of alcohol dependence can still be confirmed without these subjective control criteria being satisfied (Epstein, 2001).

Although the ADS marked an important shift away from "loss-of-control" to impaired control, Edwards & Gross (1976) questioned whether this was truly intermittent loss of self-control, or rather "*one of deciding not to exercise control*" (p. 1060), another fundamental issue which will be discussed later (see Chapter 8, on the nature of impaired self-control).

The case in support of the relevance of a research focus on subjective control over appetitive behaviour was most strongly expressed by Heather et al. (1993), who considered impaired self-control to be the defining psychological construct of the addictive behaviours. Heather et al. (1993) recognised the problems and findings of previous psychometric research and reasoned that it was due to difficulties in conceptualising self-control: Was it quantitative or non-quantitative? Was it a dichotomy, impaired control – control? Was it confined to alcoholics? Influenced in particular by the work on controlled drinking by the Sobells (e.g. Sobell & Sobell, 1976), Heather et al. argued that there was a "*need to conceptualise problems with control as a continuous variable reflecting the frequency with which episodes of impaired control occur rather than existing in an 'all or none' fashion, and this is the main advantage of speaking of impaired control rather than loss of control. It is also, of course, in keeping with modern conceptions of alcohol dependence*" (p. 701).

The impaired control scale (ICS) of Heather et al. (1993) developed from this premise had three parts assessing (1) attempts to limit drinking; (2) failures to control/limit drinking and (3) respondents' beliefs about their ability to control their drinking. A single factor for each scale was the preferred solution for the ICS. Factor analyses in subsequent validation studies (Heather et al., 1998; Marsh et al., 2002) have supported a single-factor solution for each part of the ICS and generally confirmed the reliability of the measure. Marsh et al. (2002) reaffirmed the significance of the measure in facilitating research into impaired control as a separate construct, as originally identified by Heather et al. (1993), but did not speculate on the reasons why such research has not developed during the intervening decade.

The Development of the Scale of Gambling Choices

The first attempt to assess psychometrically subjective control in gambling behaviour as an attribute independent of a mental disorder was the study of Baron et al. (1995). The study of Heather et al. (1993) was the model for this, and the items of the final version of their psychometric instrument, the Scale of Gambling Choices (SGC), were almost identical to the ICS. Following the example set in the alcoholism literature, Baron et al. (1995) assumed that subjective control was a continuous and quantitative psychological attribute: impairment

Table 2.1. *Factor analysis of national 1991 survey data*

Item	Factors				
	I	II	III	IV	h2
1. I have found it difficult to limit how much I gamble	0.85	0.22	0.18	−0.15	0.82
2. Once I have started gambling I have an irresistible urge to continue	0.74	0.20	0.04	0.36	0.72
3. When I have been near a club/hotel, totalisator agency board (TAB) or casino I have found it difficult to resist gambling	0.73	0.24	0.21	−0.12	0.64
4. Even for a single day I have found it difficult to resist gambling	0.68	0.26	0.05	0.25	0.65
5. I have been able to stop gambling before I spent all cash on me	−0.67	0.43	0.27	−0.03	0.75
6. When I have made up my mind not to gamble I have kept to it	−0.65	0.52	0.21	0.09	0.75
7. I have been able to stop gambling before the last race, TAB, club, hotel or casino closed	−0.63	0.51	0.05	0.04	0.66
8. I have been able to stop easily after a few games or bets	−0.55	0.40	0.22	−0.20	0.55
9. I have been able to gamble less often when I have wanted to	0.05	0.78	0.00	0.06	0.62
10. I have been able to stop gambling before I got into debt	−0.03	0.77	−0.02	0.05	0.60
11. When I have wanted to I could stop gambling for a week or more	0.03	0.77	−0.04	0.09	0.60
12. I have been able to resist the opportunity to start gambling	0.22	0.68	−0.17	0.12	0.55
13. When I have wanted to I have been able to cut down (gamble less) when I wanted to	−0.01	0.59	0.06	−0.31	0.44
14. I have started gambling even after deciding not to	0.14	−0.02	0.67	0.01	0.47
15. I have found myself gambling more than most people I know	−0.09	−0.08	0.65	0.09	0.44
16. Even when I only intended gambling a few dollars, I ended up gambling much more	−0.19	0.05	0.57	−0.03	0.37
17. I have started gambling even when I knew it would cause me problems (work/family/friends)	0.21	−0.04	0.45	0.13	0.23
18. I have gambled even when I knew I had an important reason not to spend money on gambling	0.07	0.08	0.30	0.45	0.31
Eigenvalue:	4.27	3.58	1.73	0.64	
% explained:	23.7	19.9	9.7	3.5	
Cumulative % explained:	23.7	43.7	53.3	56.9	

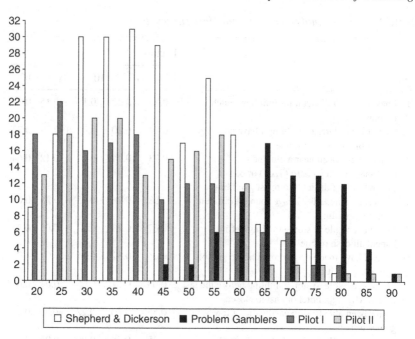

Figure 2.2. Frequency distribution of scores on the SGC (SGC: 18-item version).

Shepherd & Dickerson (2001)
☐ Regular Gaming Machine Players New South Wales (NSW) ($N = 226$,
   males $= 140$, females $= 86$, $SD = 13.27$, $M = 40.87$)
Pilot I: Haw & Dickerson (2005)*
■ Regular Gaming Machine Players NSW
Problem Gamblers
■ Problem Gamblers Attending Treatment NSW ($N = 81$; $SD = 10.03$, $M = 68.70$)
Pilot II: Haw & Dickerson (2005)**
☐ Regular Gaming Machine Players NSW

* Pilot Study 1: Participants *were recruited from seven gaming venues in Sydney,
Australia; 145 regular EGM players. There were 75 men and 70 women, with 33.8%
aged between 18 and 35, 37.9% aged between 35 and 55 and 28.3% aged over 55.
Their mean playing days per week was 2.95 (SD = 1.54), their median playing time
per playing day was 120 min (range = 10–420) and their mean dollars spent per
playing day was 41.27 (SD = 24.78). There were 15 participants (10.3%) who
reported never experiencing impaired control over the past 6 months.*
** Pilot Study 2: Participants *were recruited from two gaming venues in Sydney, 154
regular EGM players were recruited. There were 78 men and 76 women, with 48.4%
aged between 18 and 35, 26.8% aged between 35 and 55 and 24.8% aged over 55.
Their median playing days per week was 2 (range = 1–7), their median playing*

was assumed to range from complete loss of control, to frequent, to occasional, to none at all. Subjective control over gambling was defined in terms of being able to consistently maintain preferred levels of expenditure of time and money.

A set of 18 items was initially drafted, as shown in Table 2.1. Item response methodology adopted the Likert (1932) design of summated ratings, with the categories of "never", "rarely", "sometimes", "often" and "always" scored 1, 2, 3, 4 and 5, respectively. As in the ICS (Heather et al., 1993), this methodology was employed to assess the frequency with which the respondent engaged in the behaviour referred to in each item.

Baron et al. (1995) used the statistically strong sampling design of a random, stratified door knock across (1) the Australian cities of Sydney, Melbourne, Brisbane and Adelaide (287 regular gamblers and 100 diagnosed pathological gamblers) and (2) in both Western Australia and Tasmania (499 regular gamblers). Factor analyses were the main method of evaluation. The first study was not factorially interpretable, with heavy cross-loadings of some items, but from the second study the authors were able to extract three factors similar to those of the ICS.

Factor Structure: The scale yielded a three factor structure interpreted as: "*the ability to control gambling*" (represented by items 1–8), "*the intention to limit gambling*" (represented by items 9–13) and "*failure to control gambling*" (represented by items 14–18).

Correlations between the item totals of the SGC and the south oaks gambling screen (SOGS) were conducted for both samples as a method of establishing criterion validity. Large and statistically significant correlations were found for both sets of data ($r = 0.87, p < 0.001; r = 0.92, p < 0.001$) (Figure 2.2).

Baron et al. (1995) were concerned that the resultant factor solution of the SGC was in part a function of a cluster of items that were positively framed. Heather et al. (1998) encountered similar problems for the ICS sub-scale describing beliefs in ability to limit drinking. Recent research (O'Connor & Dickerson, 2003; Kyngdon, 2004) has re-examined the item set of the SGC and concluded that a 12-item (i.e. excluding items 7, 14–18), single-factor solution provides a better measure of impaired control of gambling behaviour.

Kyngdon (2004) used both factor analysis and the Rasch model for ordered response categories to psychometrically explore the structure of the SGC.

Caption for fig. 2.2 (*cont.*).
time per playing day was 120 min (range = 10–600 min) and their median dollars spent per playing day was 50 (range = 5–1500). There were seven participants (4.5%) who reported never experiencing impaired control over the past 6 months and 40.9% scored of five or more on the SOGS.

Respondents ($N = 210$) were recruited to represent a range of frequency of usage of mainly gaming machines, from occasional to regular, and included a clinical sample of problem gamblers attending counselling services. Participants completed the full version of the SGC (i.e. the original 18-item scale). The results of the item response theory (IRT) using the Rasch model provided a basis for concluding that the 12-item version was able to measure the "single, relevant dimension of control" suggested by the factor analysis: factor loadings after Varimax rotation confirmed the original concerns of Baron et al. (1995) that the factor structure was a function of the item wording and order of presentation.

Independent Confirmation of the Dimension of Self-control of Gambling Behaviour

The development of the SGC described above followed very closely the work of Heather et al. (1993) for the ICS, and assumed that self-control varied along a quantitative dimension that included no impairment, to significant effort to maintain control, to frequent impaired control of gambling behaviour. Kyngdon (2003) in seeking to consolidate the potential significance of subjective control to the addictions generally, identified the need to explore alternative methods of measurement, ones that did not assume that it was quantifiable or that it had a particular dimensional structure, and also that overcame the well-documented limitations of factor analysis (Wright, 1996).

Kyngdon (2003; and full report of study summarised below at Kyngdon & Dickerson, 2005) completed empirical studies with scales constructed using a method called "ordinal determinable" (Michell, 1994, 1998), evaluated within the conceptual frame of "unfolding theory" (Coombs, 1950, 1964). The Subjective Control scale of control over urges to engage in gambling behaviour was designed together with two other similar scales to parallel the content of the SGC (Baron et al., 1995). After rigorous pilot testing the scale was as follows.

The Subjective Control Scale of Control Over Urges to Gamble

(A) *I am free to gamble at my leisure as it does not cause any problems and I never experience strong impulses to gamble.*

(B) *I sometimes experience strong impulses to gamble, but I can easily resist them without any conscious effort and my gambling does not cause any problems.*

(C) *I sometimes feel strong impulses to gamble and while easily resisted, it does take some conscious effort; but my gambling does not cause any problems.*

(D) *I often have strong impulses to gamble that are difficult to resist, but not very difficult, and my gambling causes few but only minor problems.*

(E) *The strong impulses to gamble I often have are very difficult, but not impossible, to resist even though my gambling causes several problems.*

(F) *My frequent, strong impulses to gamble are impossible to resist and my gambling causes several, significant problems that are very distressing.*

Participant groups ranged from infrequent gamblers, regular electronic gaming machine (EGM) players recruited in venues and a clinical group of diagnosed pathological gamblers. Measures included the SOGS (Lesieur & Blume, 1987), the SGC (Baron et al., 1995) and measures of the level of involvement in gambling.

The Subjective Control scale results revealed a unidimensional, unfolded quantitative J scale that is a common or dominant pathway/ordering of the scale items (only 3% of the individual (I) scales fell outside). The same dominant pathway was confirmed at retest and concurrent validity with the 12-item SGC (O'Connor & Dickerson, 2003) was 0.82 (0.83 on retest). Interestingly *two* discernible factors emerged from both test and retest data accounting for 73% and 72% of the variance respectively: findings consistent with the *extra factor phenomenon* (Coombs & Kao, 1960; Coombs, 1964, 1975). (Very similar results were obtained for the other two scales: see Kyngdon, 2003.)

Kyngdon & Dickerson (2005) concluded that the results supported the assumption of a continuous quantifiable dimension of self-control from effortless choice to significant impaired control of gambling behaviour: a dimension common to all three groups of, infrequent, regular and pathological gamblers. In speculating on the merits of applying the same methods to problem drinking, where the use of factor analysis as the main method in developing the ADS may have contributed to the less than central role currently played by impaired control, it was noted that: *"Edwards (1986) encouraged the examination of subjective control as an attribute independent of the ADS, but he did so by extolling the use of factor analysis. The results of the present study, however, cast strong doubt upon factor analysis being a genuine method of psychological measurement. It may be the case that because factor analysis has been used to such an extent in relation to the ADS that not all genuinely unidimensional attributes relevant to addiction to alcohol have been identified. Single dimensions may have been 'split' into two ostensibly separate dimensions: that is the two factor phenomenon (Coombs & Kao, 1960; Coombs, 1964, 1975) as demonstrated in the present study"* (Kyngdon & Dickerson, 2005, p. 11).

In the present context of reviewing the measurement of self-control of gambling behaviour, the work of Kyngdon (2003) provided fundamental support for studying self-control of gambling as a quantifiable dimension in its own right, rather than as part or a subset of harmful impacts or diagnostic criteria of problem/pathological gambling.

A Qualitative Study of Self-control in Youth Gamblers

As discussed in the previous chapter, youth gamblers aged 16–25 have been identified in prevalence surveys in some countries as having the highest risk of the harmful impacts of gambling (Gupta & Derevensky, 1998). A major concern in the critical appraisal of these results has been the reliability and validity of the measures used. One concern has arisen from the assumption made in the design of some well-established measures of youth problem gambling; that the diagnostic criteria of pathological gambling in youth will be the "same" as in adults, that the harmful impacts will be similar. The minor rewording of some of the adult DSM criteria (APA, 1994), before using them as items in surveys without independent validation, exemplifies this approach (e.g. Fisher, 2000).

Maddern (2004) adopted a methodology that made no assumptions about youth gamblers' self-control over their gambling, whether it was a concern common to all, whether it was an important aspect of their gambling, or even whether, when impaired, was a potential source of harmful impacts. Her objective was to revisit these important issues with the minimum of assumptions using a qualitative approach to data collection, but rigorous numeric analysis of the transcribed interview texts.

A sample of 34 participants, aged 16–24 years and who gambled once per week or more often on continuous forms such as gaming machines, casino table games and off-course betting ("regular gamblers", Productivity Commission, 1999), were recruited. Recruiting both from clubs and casinos, and via the networks of the interviewers on a "snow-ball" basis, interviews were completed at the preferred gambling venue of the participant (the seven under-age gamblers were interviewed in nearby coffee-bars).

The majority of the participants were single, and the male to female ratio was 3:1. Most respondents had completed year 11 or higher, and seven were currently studying. Eight were unemployed, with almost half in full-time employment; the most common occupational group was sales/clerical and incomes ranged from less than $116 per week to $1154 per week (median between $289 and $384 per week). One third of the participants spoke a language other than English and lived across 27 different suburbs of southern and western metropolitan Sydney.

Semi-structured interviews were completed, ranging in duration from 20 min to 1 h and 45 min (in to over 70 h of transcribed text). The interview opened with the question, "Can you tell me about your life? What is it like, the good things and the bad things?".... A single prompt of "Can you tell me more?" was used. (This scene-setting question was transcribed and coded separately and used in a developmental study presented in Chapter 3.)

The interview then proceeded with eight questions about gambling:

1. Are any of the good or bad things (i.e. in your life) because of your gambling?
2. Does gambling jeopardise your goals in any way?
3. If you want to win at gambling what is the best thing you could do?
4. Have you ever had a big win/loss?
5. Can you think about the last time you spent a "lot" of money gambling?
6. When you have been gambling how do you stop?
7. Do you ever feel any conflict about gambling-like one part of you says "yes" and another part says "no"?
8. Is there anything else we have not asked you about gambling that you would like to say or think is important?

The study, in the tradition of Grounded Theory, was true to the iterative process of empirically driven theory generation. Data analysis was undertaken with repeated passes through the data using NUD*IST version 4 (Richards & Richards, 1997).

The emerging "Limit Maintenance Model" examined themes supportive and detrimental to self-control under two key areas, limit setting and emotional responses, and validated the groups emerging on the basis of their styles of control against the reported harmful impacts of gambling (Maddern, 2004). The latter were taken from the text of each participant and scored using the Harms scale of the "Harmful impacts of gambling" used in the national survey in Australia by the Productivity Commission (1999) (Figure 2.3).

Three types of limit setting were established:

1. No specific limits ($N = 3$).
2. Target limits ($N = 12$, plus $N = 5$ who revise limits once only).
3. Contingency limits: continually revising or setting vague or broad limits ($N = 14$).

No Specific Limits (N = 3)

The first group described finishing their gambling sessions without having any specific time or money limit in mind: they rarely spent more than they were comfortable with and did not find it difficult to end a session; it occurred when

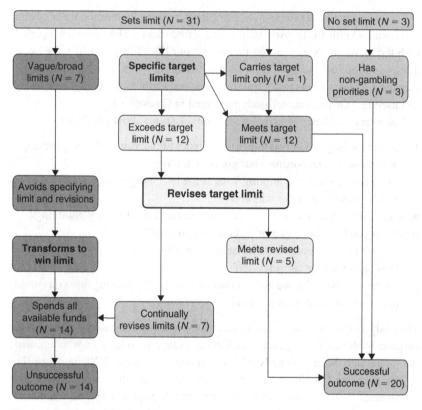

Figure 2.3. The limit maintenance model (Maddern, 2004).

they had reached a point when the decision was a natural part of choosing to go elsewhere, to accompany/meet a friend, because they were bored etc. In interview, when looking back on their gambling, each was able to specify the expenditure limit they would apply, and for each this was well within their financial means. None reported any ambivalence about wanting to continue gambling and needing to prevent further losses/expenditure.

This small sub-group of regular young gamblers provided an important anchor point for the model: Maddern (2004) argued that the apparent absence of goals did not mean that their behaviour was directionless, but rather was evidence of an absence of processing at a conscious cognitive level and was dynamic self-regulation, Pintrich (2000). There was no evidence that these three gamblers depended on external regulation to control their gambling; it was autonomous Grolnick & Ryan (1987). Further evidence for this interpretation was provided by the absence of any gambling related negative emotional states reported by these gamblers. Thus Maddern suggested that the autonomous self-regulation of gambling might be protective against dysphoric mood because a goal is achieved, that is pleasure and entertainment without any harmful impacts, and these outcomes accord with personal values.

Target Limits (N = 12, plus N = 5 who revise limits once only)

Twelve participants pre-set and consistently met their expenditure limits. They differed from the "no specific limits" group reporting conscious monitoring of expenditure throughout the gambling session, regularly considered the "costs" of exceeding their limits, and were able to coherently articulate the reasons (e.g. self-knowledge of feeling uncomfortable owing money, not paying essential bills etc.). Occasionally when limits were exceeded, respondents in this group viewed the lapse within its specific circumstances and how they were feeling at the time, rather than as an indication of a general inability to apply limits.

Included in this group, who typically successfully met their limits, were five respondents who described exceeding their initial limit and then revising their limit once only to enable them to play longer. This reset limit was met and the session stopped.

Contingency Limits: Continually Revising or Setting Vague or Broad Limits (N = 14)

This group of regular players was typified by an inability to achieve and stick to their preferred levels of time and cash expenditure on gambling. Half could specify a cash limit for a session and then continually revised this as each limit was exceeded: a session typically ended when all limits were exceeded or all cash-in-hand was spent. Ending the session was associated with emotional ambivalence, conflicting motives and goals, and a breakdown in the self-regulation process. These players had little confidence in their ability to stick to their limits and control their expenditure on gambling.

There were seven regular gamblers, all young men, who avoided the negative emotional impact of continually failing to meet specific limits by adopting what Maddern called "the manner of entrepreneurs engaged in a business deal"; limits were reframed in terms of preferred levels of winning before ending the session. As with all preferred gaming machine play, planning to achieve such goals is illusory, but in the short term such a strategy may be emotionally protective. In terms of self-regulatory processes, these players no longer monitored their expenditure, and in terms of personal values, continuing to gamble and to be seen as a winner was preferred, despite large losses and debts.

The emerging Limit Maintenance Model was then re-examined in the context of reported emotions and harmful impacts of gambling. Groups 1 and 2 were taken together as evidencing the ability to self-regulate, and then compared with Group 3, the contingency regulated players.

Emotions and the Ability to Self-regulate Gambling

It was common for all participants to associate stressful life events, both episodic and chronic, with impairment of control over gambling involvement. The self-regulated respondents were aware that specific events that triggered emotions were often the cause of occasional excessive gambling: there was an understanding of how the negative emotions, notably guilt and emotion, had precipitated the desire to gamble, or how gambling had been used to relieve such feelings. This awareness in those who self-regulated their gambling was also linked to planned preventative strategies such as only taking a limited sum of cash to a venue knowing, that under such emotional constraints, they were at risk.

In contrast, the contingency regulated group were significantly less able to articulate any connections between life event stressors/emotions and their gambling. In fact there was a tendency to attribute their feelings of guilt and depression to their excessive gambling. This failure to accurately attribute their feeling to life event stressors other than gambling, was associated with the belief that they were quite unable to control their expenditure on gambling; typically events interceded such as the loss of all cash on hand or the venue closing.

Reported Harmful Impacts and the Ability to Self-regulate

The reported harmful impacts occurring in the texts of each participant were extracted and scored according to the Harm scale used by the Productivity Commission (1999). As shown in Table 2.2, the self-regulated group were less likely to report such personal "costs" of their gambling, particularly the more severe impacts. This matches the known strong positive relationship between the measure of impaired control over gambling (SGC) and measures of the harmful impacts of gambling such as the SOGS and the victorian gambling scale (VGS) (Baron et al., 1995; O'Connor et al., 2005). Maddern also concluded that the order in which the harmful impacts occurred were the same for both groups, with money concerns first being reported, followed by gambling

Table 2.2. *Summary of harms by level of self-control (adapted from Maddern, 2004)*

Harm category	Self-regulated ($N = 20$) (%)	Contingency regulated ($N = 14$) (%)
Money	45	100
Mood	35	79
Relationship conflict	15	57
Career		29
Self (intrapersonal)		29
Possessions and defaults		21
Broken relationships		14
Criminal acts to support gambling		14

related dysphoria, and that these two were common to most regular young gamblers.

In the present context this qualitative study illustrated that the interview responses to one question out of the eight, "When you have been gambling how do you stop?" proved to be a central coordinating theme to participants' diverse experiences of gambling, linking styles of control with negative emotions and the likelihood of gambling resulting in harmful impacts. It suggests that the impaired self-control commonly observed and measured in adult regular gamblers, and now detailed in 16–24 year old men and women who have chosen to gamble regularly on continuous forms, is a phenomenon that develops relatively rapidly in the first few years.

The Relationship Between Impaired Control and Chasing

"Chasing", the attempt to recover ones gambling losses by further gambling, has a central position in explanations of pathological gambling (e.g. *The Chase*, Lesieur, 1984) and is a common diagnostic criteria (DSM-IV, APA 1994: item A6, see Table 1.2, Chapter 1). Chasing has been studied in experimental settings (e.g. Breen & Zuckerman, 1999) but only recently has there been an examination of its characteristics and an empirical study of the conditions under which it takes place (O'Connor et al., 1995; O'Connor & Dickerson, 1997, 2003a). In the present context, the main issue is whether chasing is an integral component of impairment of self-control over gambling, or whether it is a separate distinguishable factor contributing to the harmful impacts.

Earlier work, although limited by the use of a single item measure of chasing embedded in a survey of bettors recruited in an off-course venue (Dickerson et al., 1987), illustrated the question: of the mainly regular gamblers, 30% were found to occasionally chase and another 14% usually or always chased their losses. Chasing was related to staying to listen or watch the race (i.e. continuous gambling), making bet selections in the venue, last minute bet placement, last minute changes to selection, spending more than planned and attempts to reduce or stop betting. The conclusion drawn was that chasing is a *"central characteristic of a complex of experiences and behaviours that are concerned with the subjective control of gambling behaviour"* (p. 678).

Prior to the sequence of studies by O'Connor, the majority of the work into chasing had been of an ethnographic nature (e.g. Lesieur, 1984; Rosecrance, 1986; Browne, 1989), providing ecologically valid insights but not permitting the detailed, quantitative analysis of its relationship with other variables. Following a careful qualitative exploration of gamblers' definitions of chasing and the piloting of a measure of chasing that included three psychological aspects, cognitive/behavioural intention to chase, emotional/urges to chase and behavioural (actually chasing) (O'Connor et al., 1995; O'Connor & Dickerson, 1997), a community-based survey of regular off-course gamblers and EGM players was completed which included the SGC (12-item version), levels of gambling involvement and demographic information (O'Connor & Dickerson, 2003a).

The measure of chasing used in this study assessed the reported frequency of the three psychological aspects of chasing under the following conditions:

1. Heavy losses, large wins and near-misses, replicated across,
2. Chasing *within a session* for example "Have you tried to get back your losses before the end of a session? and *across sessions*, "Have you returned at a later time or date to try and win back past losses?".

These different conditions were essential to develop a better understanding of chasing, the former in challenging/controlling for the clinical and ethnographic observation that chasing occurred after **losses**, and the latter sustaining a long held distinction made in the alcohol field (Jellinek, 1960; Heather, 1991).

Chasing was found to be a common feature of regular gambling and there was strong support for conceptualising it as a constellation of cognitive, emotional (urges) and behavioural components associated with continuing to gamble and with increasing the size of stakes. The reported frequency of chasing was very similar for both win and loss contexts. (The results detailing the different components of chasing are further discussed in Chapter 3 in the sections on emotional and cognitive variables that influence self-control.)

The key findings in relation to the SGC measure of impaired control were as follows:

- All components of chasing, for both forms of gambling and for men and women in the EGM group, were strongly correlated with the SGC and with the traditional single item measures of chasing.
- Increasing the size of bets after a near miss was the item most strongly associated with impaired control (SGC) for the off-course betting gamblers.
- Gamblers who returned later to chase had significantly higher SGC scores than those who only chased within sessions.

Although this project requires further research before firm conclusions may be drawn, it appears that chasing is an integral component of the experience of impaired self-control reported by regular consumers of continuous forms of gambling, a group known to be most at risk of the harmful impacts of gambling (Productivity Commission, 1999). It raises two distinct but not mutually exclusive possibilities:

1. That a measure of impaired control should include items that assess chasing within and between sessions: such a scale might be a stronger predictor of the harmful impacts of gambling.
2. That the cognitive aspects of chasing are like other cognitive themes such as a belief in skill and control over chance-determined events, and therefore a secondary process to the primary process that erodes self-control (i.e. conditioning rewarded by strong positive emotional experiences). In the following chapter, the possibility that gambling cognitions contribute to impaired control by providing a post hoc "self-explanation" of excessive involvement is examined further.

Impaired Control and Different Forms of Gambling

In the previous chapter it was concluded that problem gambling can arise from a selective preference for the consumption of one specific form or product, especially if the preferred form is a continuous type such a EGM play, off-course betting or casino table games: within the same individual problem gambler non-preferred forms, even if regularly consumed, such as lottery tickets, may not contribute actively to the harmful impacts, and may present no problems of control over time and money expenditure. Thus very similar addictive pictures of harmful impacts may arise from the regular involvement in very different gambling processes. The problem gambler who prefers EGM play will be seated in relative privacy at a machine playing games at the rate of 13 per minute with a period of 3 seconds between staking and the outcome being revealed on the screen (Haw, 2000). In contrast, the other most popular continuous form of gambling in Australia for men, horse/dog racing, involves selecting, writing out a bet and placing a stake on average every 2–3 min. The period between stake and race outcome ranges from just under one to several minutes, and even longer when stewards call an inquiry into the results.

If these very different gambling processes are implicated in the erosion of self-control, and ultimately in the cause of the harmful impacts, then the very different structural characteristics and related gambling behaviours provide a research opportunity to establish which are the necessary conditions to facilitate an addictive process. For example, does the possibly greater subjective arousal experienced during off-course betting "support" the longer and variable time cycle compared to EGM play (Dickerson, 1991)?

Thus the question addressed by O'Connor and Dickerson (2003) was whether two such very different gambling processes are associated with a common, generic process of impaired control.

The shortened 12-item version of the SGC was used with samples of venue recruited regular gamblers who preferred off-course betting (TAB) (84 men) and gaming machine play (EGM) (73 women and 64 men). There were no differences between the EGM and TAB samples on employment status, income, marital status, education levels or country of origin, and there was overall a reasonable match with Australian demographic patterns (Australian Bureau of Statistics (ABS), 1997). Expenditure on gambling, both net and as a proportion of income, and gambling debts did not distinguish between TAB and EGM gamblers. TAB gamblers spent more time gambling than EGM players and women EGM players spent more time gambling per week than men.

The SGC scores did not differ significantly between the EGM and TAB gambler groups, and the preferred factor structure from principal component analysis was a similar, single factor, structure (for a detailed discussion see O'Connor, 2000). Higher scores of impaired control were strongly associated with greater gambling involvement, time and money expenditure, and gambling debts.

The authors concluded that impaired control appears a valid concept with face, construct and concurrent validity. The generic nature of impaired control was demonstrated by the lack of differences in the total scores on the SGC for the two very different forms of gambling, the very similar factor structure for each group of gamblers, and the absence of a gender difference in reported impaired control within the EGM sample. This result was expected given the much earlier survey results summarised in Corless & Dickerson (1989) that included data from regular patrons of off-course betting in the UK and Australia as well as reports from regular EGM players in social clubs in Australia. Nonetheless, O'Connor and Dickerson's (2003) results were the first to provide psychometric confirmation of the similar high levels of impaired self-control experienced by regular gamblers who preferred, and were currently involved in, different forms of continuous gambling.

Progress in the Measurement and Definition of Impaired Control of Gambling Behaviour

Priority must be given to the work of Kyngdon (2003) drawing on methods and theory from mathematical psychology and whose results provided fundamental and compelling evidence that self-control of gambling is:

- A dimension from free effortless enjoyment of gambling through increasing effort to resist impulses to gamble, to limit time, to maintain control*, to a point where frequent impulses cannot be resisted and self-control cannot be maintained.
- A dimension that is quantifiable with its properties sustained across the full range of gambling involvement from infrequent, to regular gamblers to pathological/problem gamblers.

The scales used by Kyngdon include two key definitional components of impaired control over gambling, an awareness of problems arising from gambling and attempts to resist urges/excess. In the "pathways model" Blaszczynski & Nower (2002) *specified "repeated unsuccessful attempts to resist the urge in the context of a genuine desire to cease, as the central, diagnostic and foundational feature of pathological gambling"* (p. 488). This leaves the fraught question of whether attempts at control, as assessed by the scales, were in the context of a genuine desire to cease. Such a question goes to the heart of the nature of self-control in the addictions and is not readily addressed using psychometric measures. The fact that the clinical group of pathological gamblers, who were attending for therapy/intervention and might therefore reasonably be assumed to be genuinely motivated at least to reduce their gambling, gave the same dominant J scale solution goes some way to addressing this aspect of the definition.

The issue raised by Blaszczynski & Nower's (2002) is that the impaired self-control experienced by pathological gamblers, that plays a central, causal role in their mental disorder, is qualitatively different from the impairment experienced by regular gamblers. The results for the measurement of impaired self-control presented and discussed above tend to contradict such a view: self-control over gambling appears to be a continuum.

(* *Note*: Only the impulse scale was detailed above: the two other Subjective Control scales, limiting of time gambling and general control of gambling scales gave similar results – Kyngdon, 2003.)

The SGC 12-item

The recent factor and item analysis (Kyngdon, 2004) confirmed that the 12-item version of the SGC is the preferred traditional psychometric method: *"The overall congruence of the factor analytic and IRT findings suggest that a genuine factor was indeed assessed by these 12-items ... all 12-items are assessing one relevant dimension only. This could be termed "general ability to control gambling"* (p. 176). The single relevant dimension was evidenced by similar item characteristic curves for each item across three groups of participants representing levels of involvement in gambling from infrequent to pathological/problem gambling.

O'Connor & Dickerson (2003) also confirmed a single-factor structure for the 12-item version (accounting for 60% of the variance); this structure held for two different types of regular, continuous gambling, off-course betting and EGM play (when a second factor for EGM play was interpreted as an artefact of a low response rate on two items), and for both men and women players.

Reliability

The internal consistency of the SGC is generally high (e.g. 0.97, as measured by the person separation index (PSI): Kyngdon, 2004; alpha 0.92, O'Connor & Dickerson, 2003) and test-retest over a 6-month period gave a correlation of 0.67 although as described later in Chapter 4, this was in the context of almost 20% of the regular gamblers significantly changing their level of reported impaired control (O'Connor et al., 2005).

Validity

The SGC correlates positively and moderately with measures of involvement in gambling for different types of regular gambling (O'Connor & Dickerson, 2003; O'Connor et al., 2005). The original SGC (18-items) correlated very highly with the SOGS (0.87 and 0.92: Baron et al., 1995) and the 12-item scale correlated 0.83 (and 0.82 at 6-month retest) with the VGS (Ben-Tovim et al., 2001). Thus high scores on the SGC are indicative of significant deleterious consequences arising from gambling whether these effects are measured in terms of the likelihood of mental disorder, pathological gambling, or in terms of harm to the individual player and their family.

3

Impaired Control and its Relationship to other Variables Implicated in the Development of Pathological Gambling

Initial Thoughts on Modelling Impaired Self-Control: Key Variables

Cornish's (1978) influential review of gambling proposed that a person's initial choice of a gambling product was a function of a variety of factors including availability, prior knowledge from parental gambling and serendipity. The opportunity to *sample* a wide range of gambling products might today be added for those jurisdictions where most gambling products are legalised. Cornish envisaged that the change, should it occur, to regular consumption of a particular form of gambling, was associated with a process of person–product adaptations as the individual learnt to use the gambling to satisfy current needs.

In this chapter the primary focus remains on regular gamblers, and in selecting psychological variables that may contribute to the process of maintaining or losing control, we have not considered the factors that may determine a person's initial choice of gambling product. It must be accepted that some of the variables that influence this "first" choice may also be significant in determining the extent to which an individual experiences impaired control over their gambling. An obvious example is when parental modelling by a problem gambler may not only determine both their child's choice of gambling product, but also their level of self-control over how much they gamble.

A Developmental Perspective on Impaired Control of Gambling

There is evidence that problem gamblers may start their involvement with gambling during adolescence, sometimes as young as 9 or 10 years of age (Custer, 1982; Derevensky et al., 1996; Wynne et al., 1996), raising concerns about their long-term well-being. Although changes in the legal availability of gambling would be expected to be a confounding factor, there is evidence that a key variable is the role that family members may play. Studies have shown a link between parental gambling and that of their children (Jacobs et al., 1989; Lesieur et al., 1991). Oei & Raylu (2003) suggest that there are essentially two components, *genetic* (Comings et al., 1996; Eisen et al., 1998; Winters & Rich, 1998) and *social learning* (Gupta & Derevensky, 1997; Hardoon & Derevensky, 2002), and they provided some evidence for the latter when illustrating the similarity of gambling cognitions and behaviours for parents and children in 185 family units.

In the qualitative study of youth gamblers by Maddern (2004), reported in the previous chapter, the ability of the respondents to set and maintain gambling limits was discussed in terms of the degree to which the gambling behaviour was externally initiated and controlled versus self-initiated and managed. The latter was considered intrinsically motivated (Deci & Ryan, 1985), limits were set and adhered to, conveying the sense of personal agency consistent with truly autonomous behaviour (Kuhl, 1992). In contrast the control exercised by the contingency-regulated gamblers was coercive; they were pressured by the feelings and circumstances of the moment and this was associated with reporting of more frequent and intense harmful impacts arising from their gambling than for the self-regulated gamblers. Maddern argued that the developmental skills available to each youth gambler would relate both to their style of self-control and their coping with the harmful impacts.

Psychosocial Maturity, Self-Regulation and Reported Harmful Impacts of Gambling

"Autonomy" was selected by Maddern as a broad developmental theme common to both self-regulation and developmental theories, the Eriksonian conceptualisation preferred primarily because there existed a valid and reliable measure of Erikson's stages of development based on content analysis (Content Analysis Scales of Psychosocial Maturity (CASPM); Viney et al., 1995).

The data for the analysis was provided by the texts ($N = 34$) of the participants' responses to the first interview question, "I'd like you to talk to me for a few minutes about what life is like at the moment – the good things and the bad – what is it like for you?" The majority of participants did not mention gambling during this stage of the interview and the text of these responses was not included in the development of the Limit Maintenance Model.

Typed transcripts were prepared from the taped responses and readied for content analysis by dividing them into clauses each with an active verb. Analysis and scoring followed the standard procedures for the CASPM (Viney et al., 2001). An independent, blind rater scored 10 of the 34 interview responses to this first question achieving a reliability coefficient of alpha = 0.83.

Activity on the developmental dimensions, indicated by the greatest number of scored clauses was found for Trust/Mistrust, Autonomy/Constraint, Initiative/ Hesitancy, Industry/Inferiority and Affinity/Isolation. The self-regulated gamblers scored higher than the contingency-regulated gamblers on each of these dimensions except Industry/Hesitancy. For both groups the most active constructs were Affinity/Isolation and Autonomy/Constraint, the former suggesting that forging warm, reciprocal and satisfactory relationships was the most important developmental process occurring for respondents in this sample of youth, and the latter that managing issues of choice, freedom and self-control was also a significant focus in their lives.

The only significant correlation between an emergent pole of a developmental dimension and the level of reported harmful impacts of gambling was between Autonomy and lower levels of harm (-0.33, $p < 0.05$). Maddern (2004) concluded that these results gave support to the link between psychosocial development and the likelihood of regular youth gamblers becoming problem players: *"Generally higher scores on psychosocial constructs, combined with the ability to set and maintain limits were indicative of a stable and manageable gambling pattern."* (p. 185), but tempered with, *"Resolving psychosocial skills positively did not entirely prevent gambling problems, it did however buffer the severity of the problem and would be likely to facilitate a speedy recovery with a relatively intact sense of self"* (p. 186).

The results of this first developmental study of youth gamblers provide some support for the approach that forms the main story line to this monograph, namely that research into the addictive aspects of gambling may benefit from "separating" problem/pathological gambling into impaired self-control and the harmful impacts. Different psychological resources or skills may be involved in the processes that modify each of the outcomes. Despite the limitations imposed by the selection of any one particular theoretical account of psychological development, advantages accrue when the results are considered within the context of the particular theoretical model. Thus within the Ericksonion stage model:

"When Autonomy is under-developed, particularly for a youthful cohort, the result is likely to be detrimental to attempting and resolving other developmental stages. Completing education and beginning a career requires a high level of Autonomy, and when Autonomy is under-developed and impaired control of gambling is added to the mix, the adverse effects are multiplied. Respondents whose self-concept was dominated by constraint felt that their choices in life were limited . . . they had no alternative but to spend all their money on gambling." (Maddern, 2004, p. 182)

From a psychological perspective, the research by Maddern is both intuitively and conceptually more appropriate to the study of youth gamblers than the use of measures adapted from the definition of an adult mental disorder, pathological gambling.

The Key Variables in Modelling Impaired Control

Gambling Involvement

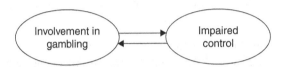

In the earlier position article (Dickerson & Baron, 2000), it was pointed out that there is an inevitable circularity between impaired control and how often and how long a person gambles: *"the more a person gambles the greater the opportunity to lose control and the more a person experiences impaired control the more they gamble"* (p. 1150). The reports of professional gamblers (Allcock & Dickerson, 1986) suggest that there is an increased risk of impaired control arising from increased involvement per se and professional gamblers, aware that they typically gamble more often and with larger stakes than others, adopt strategies that aid control, such as detailed accounting and bet selection systems.

Moving beyond the frame of impaired control to the broader picture of problem gambling, all prevalence surveys, that also assess respondents' current consumption of available gambling forms, find strong associations between frequency and expenditure on gambling and measures of pathological gambling and/or the harmful impacts of gambling (NORC, 1999; Productivity Commission, 1999).

The relative strength of the two pathways, involvement on impaired control and vice versa, is important not just from a theoretical model building perspective but also from a policy and harm minimisation perspective: if the former is the main driver of impaired control then changes to ease of access, marketing or changes to make forms of gambling "safer" might be the preferred emphasis for harm reduction. If impaired control is driven primarily by other psychological variables, such as individual differences, prior mood, etc., then the contemporary focus on assisting the individual gambler to maintain self-control and gamble in a low-risk manner, might be preferred.

In the "pathways model" the interaction between level of involvement in gambling and self-control is summarised for regular gamblers as follows:

"Principles of learning theory and cognitive processes are instrumental in fostering a loss of control for all pathological gamblers. However it is argued that there is a subset of behaviourally conditioned gamblers who at times may meet formal criteria for pathological gambling but who are characterised by an absence of any specific premorbid feature of psychopathology. Essentially these gamblers fluctuate between the realms of regular/heavy and excessive gambling because of effects of conditioning, distorted cognitions surrounding probability of winning and/or a series of bad judgements or poor decision-making rather than because of impaired control." (Blaszczynski & Nower, 2002, p. 492)

Thus both Cornish (1978), from a general psychological perspective, and Blaszczynski and Nower (2002) from a mental disorder context, place considerable emphasis on the part played by the processes of learning/conditioning as the gambler comes to regularly use a preferred product and/or use it excessively.

In the gambling literature there are several types of research that have explored how best to understand this process of change and to implicate key aspects of psychological learning theory:

1. Early attempts to explore the impact of schedules of reinforcement using mechanical slot machines in laboratory settings (Lewis & Duncan, 1958; Strickland & Grote, 1967; Levitz, 1971), none of which satisfy the research requirements detailed in the previous chapter.

2. A method designed to examine the validity of cognitive explanations of persistent and problematic gambling, the "thinking aloud" method in which the player was instructed to voice their thoughts while they gambled (e.g. Ladouceur et al., 1991; Walker, 1992a; Griffiths, 1994b). The dependent variable was a comparison of irrational to rational statements, where rational was defined, for example by Walker (1992a) " . . . *statement of strategy that is correct. . . . in relation to the game*" (p. 254). The predominance of irrational statements, especially for gaming machines where there are only a limited number of ways of saying that wins are chance determined, was never convincing, but more particularly the method was intrusive, placing an unusual demand on players and artificially increased session length (Griffiths, 1994b).

3. There have also been attempts to use observational approaches that record the behaviours, thoughts and feelings, including physiological events such as heart rates of gamblers in venues. The most successful was without doubt that of Anderson and Brown (1984), not because it informed learning

theory accounts of regular gambling, but because, as discussed earlier, it showed how laboratory studies gave not only weaker effects but also sometimes entirely artificial results. Two observational sequences of studies in Australia (Dickerson et al., 1991, 1992; Delfabbro & Winefield, 1999) recorded gaming machine play by volunteer players while gambling in venues using their preferred machine. Although both projects showed that larger reinforcement disrupted the rate of playing, and that the behaviours, including staking patterns, in regular gamblers are more stereotyped than infrequent players, the differences in methodology did not enable the conflicting results for rate of play and win size to be resolved. Haw (2000) provides a detailed and critical review of both projects and concluded that the results, " . . . *indicated that poker machine playing behaviour does not unequivocally match operant theory predictions*" (p. 132).

There are two more recent strands of research that address the question of how best to conceptualise the interaction between gamblers and the gambling sequence of events. Firstly, there are continuing international endeavours to make gaming machines "safer", to remove those structural characteristics that may encourage excess or addictive usage or to add features that maintain self-control (see Chapter 6, p. 112). Secondly, there are the first studies to be completed that place industry derived measures of player gambling, that is machine records of all games/stakes and real-time player tracking systems, in the appropriate psychological frame of reference (Haw, 2000).

The latter studies are given priority at this stage of the text as Haw's unique work reveals both the complexity of the task and provides a methodology for future research in the area. In so doing he also provides the reader with an understanding of why the current search for the "safe" gaming machine has generated such confusing results.

Level of Involvement in Gambling and Structural Characteristics

In gaming machines, schedules of reinforcement and size of reinforcement are integral components of machine design, and are the internal structural characteristics that have been the main focus of research. Since Skinner's (1953) original statement, that the gambler was like the pigeon with its five responses per second for many hours and was therefore victim of an unpredictable contingency of reinforcement, the slot machine as an example of variable ratio (VR) schedules has become a standard in most introductory psychology texts, despite clear demonstrations that gaming machines of this type operate with a random ratio (RR) of reinforcement (Hurlburt et al., 1980).

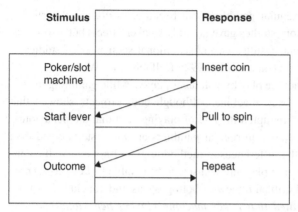

Figure 3.1. Alternating sequence of stimuli and responses available in poker machine play (until ca. 1970) (from Haw, 2000).

Haw (2000) provides an empirical example of the very different player experience that can be generated by comparable VR and RR schedules. Figures 3.1 and 3.2 are a reminder that contemporary machines of the type featured in Haw's research have a very much more complex pattern of stimulus–response than the original archetypal gaming machine, and his results must be considered in this context.

In comparing VR and RR schedules, Haw noted that VR schedules have a rectangular distribution of reinforcement and the run of non-reinforced responses is fixed and limited: for example VR 2.5, reinforcement will occur 25% of the time after one play, 25% of the time after two plays, 25% of the time after three plays and 25% of the time after four plays. In contrast the RR 2.5 schedule permits the run of non-reinforcement to be unlimited, skewing the average rate of reinforcement to a higher figure and therefore, argued Haw, the majority of reinforcement should occur closer to, and below, the mean. The hypothesis that the RR schedule will have a mode lower than the mean was tested playing a typical electronic gaming machine (EGM) in a gaming venue; a 1-cent denomination with a maximum 20 pay-lines. The "sample" was 406 games played with 20 pay-lines (stake size 20 cents) and 457 games with 10 pay-lines.

This real-life illustration shows the potential significance to player behaviour of the difference between the schedules: despite the similarity of the mean reward rates between VR 2.5 and the average for all plays on the EGM of RR 2.56, the rates under the hypothetical and each actual condition of play are very different with the 20 cents/game stake being rewarded 45% of the time compared with 28% for 10 lines/cents. Haw speculates that the early learning of

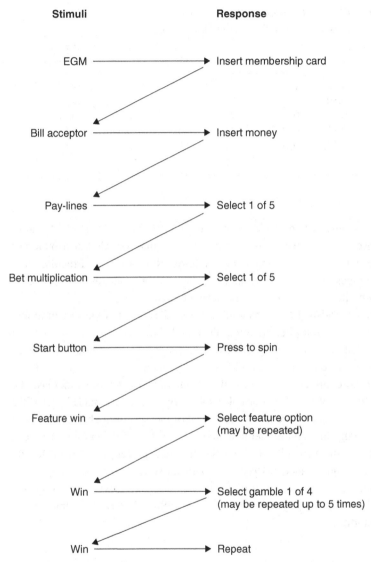

Figure 3.2. Alternating sequence of stimuli and responses available in current EGM play (from Haw, 2000).

players may be influenced by this distinct difference between the richness of the schedule for different stake size shaping the player to bet more lines, so that the typical stake on a machine, regardless of denomination, is the permitted maximum. Table 3.1, like Figure 3.2 above illustrates the complexity of the

Impaired Control and its Relationship to other Variables

Table 3.1. *Matrix of available betting responses and frequency of occurrence in EGM play (1994) (from Haw, 2000)*

	1 line	3 lines	5 lines	7 lines	9 lines	Bet total
Bet 1	4.70	1.52	9.31	2.95	41.23	59.71
Bet 2	0.50	0.28	2.94	0.52	15.39	19.63
Bet 3	0.07	0.09	0.98	0.41	8.56	10.11
Bet 5	0.11	0.06	0.43	0.12	5.83	6.55
Bet 10	0.13	0.10	0.11	0.04	3.61	3.96
Line total	5.52	2.06	13.78	4.03	74.62	

Values in per cent.

possible responses when playing a contemporary EGM and the gradual change in response/lines bet, across the matrix. The machine-recorded distribution of responses, which will to a large extent comprise the responses of regular players, encourages the speculation that the richer reinforcement arising from covering more lines shapes the response across to maximum lines.

Although Cornish (1978) was writing before the advent of the structural features such as the multiplier potential illustrated above, he argued that forms of gambling that offered a variety of staking levels and odds (he would have been referring to off-course betting and casino table games in the UK at the time) would be more attractive to potential consumers and would also increase the potential for gamblers to lose control. Similar arguments were made by Griffiths (1993b) in the first comprehensive appraisal of the structural characteristics of the UK fruit machine; multiplier potential, tokenisation, light and sound effects, artwork and name were all predicted to contribute to player persistence. Despite the predicted significance of structural characteristics in contributing to player persistence and impaired control over gambling, there were no published empirical tests of these hypotheses in the late 1990s when Haw completed two seminal studies.

Study I
If the key underlying hypothesis was that machine structural characteristics generate more expenditure over longer periods, then it would be expected that machines with these characteristics would record greater expenditure figures than those without. Haw selected for study the three multiplier characteristics that had transformed the player options on Australian gaming machines from 1988 onwards. These were denomination, pay-lines and bet multiplication for

each machine. The combined multiplier effects were defined in terms of four observed variables:

1. Denomination of the machine or the minimum cost of a game.
2. Denomination × maximum number of pay-lines.
3. Denomination × maximum bet multiplication.
4. Denomination × maximum pay-lines × maximum bet multiplication.

In a clarifying example of a machine with a multiplier potential made up of a 5-cent denomination, a maximum of 9 lines and a bet multiplier of 10, then the minimum cost per game is 5 cents; with maximum pay-lines the cost per game is 45 cents and the maximum possible cost per game is 450 cents (Haw, 2000).

Two hundred poker machines, currently in use in a convenience sample of eight gaming venues in Sydney, were "surveyed". The four, multiplier potential characteristics and the recorded average stake size, or response variable, were recorded. The median age of the machines was just over 9 months (i.e. they had novel, recently designed, features). The response variable was recorded on the hard drive of the machine and retrieved with the assistance of the gaming venue. The observed variables were visible on the cabinet of each machine.

Having transformed the data to satisfy the assumptions of multiple regression, the analysis revealed two significant predictors of average stake size; variables 2 and 3 above, the costs of maximum pay-lines, and maximum bet multiplication. The former was by far the stronger, and a separate bivariate regression revealed that the cost of maximum pay-lines was able to account for 85% of the variance in average stake size.

Haw concluded that this was the first empirical evidence of the impact of structural characteristics on the behaviour of gamblers. The importance of just one aspect of the multiplier effect suggested that the staking patterns, primarily of regular players (regular players have more frequent and longer sessions of play and account for approximately 85% of total expenditure; Dickerson et al., 1998), are highly stereotypical and determined by the machine denomination and the maximum number of pay-lines. Although it is an acceptable assumption that the aggregate machine data is derived mainly from regular players, it cannot be determined whether machines of higher denomination *attract* players with higher stake preferences or whether individual players staking patterns *change* as they change machines during a session.

In a subsequent analysis the best predictors of the variable machine profit were not the multiplier variables but the presence of a bill acceptor on a machine and machine age ("younger" machines are more profitable), both variables together accounting for almost 30% of variance in machine profitability. (As

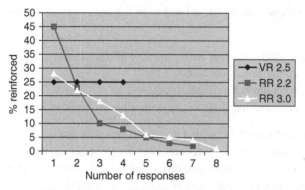

Figure 3.3. Distribution of reinforcement when playing 10 pay-lines (RR 3.0), 20 pay-lines (RR 2.2) and VR 2.5 as a hypothetical comparison.

the bill acceptor at the time was relatively new, the analysis controlled for the relationship between the predictor variables.)

Study II

In evaluating the previous results, Haw noted that the reinforcing properties of the variable denomination × maximum pay-lines were confounded and that it was not possible to establish whether the observed effect on stake size was due to the increase in size of reinforcement (associated with an increase in denomination) or the increase in frequency of the reinforcer (associated with an increase in the number of pay-lines). The latter has been illustrated in Figure 3.3 for the sample of plays under two RR schedules associated with either 10 or 20 pay-lines. Furthermore, the strength of the observed structural effect should, according to operant theory, differ between players based on their level of experience or prior learning (Chance, 1994; Catania, 1998; Mazur, 1998).

The objectives of the second study were to examine the evidence for structural effects on individual player behaviour of stake size, separating the effects of reinforcement size and frequency, and accounting for individual differences in terms of prior experience of play. In addition, in order to follow-up the results for machine profitability, it was predicted that the variable player net loss would be related to the bill acceptor and machine age.

In order to achieve these goals, a repeated measures design of player expenditure over numerous machines was required. Haw rejected the observational and video recording methods of previous studies (Dickerson et al., 1992; Delfabbro & Winefield, 1999, respectively) and for the first time used computer tracking of playing behaviour. Many of the large registered clubs in New South Wales

Table 3.2. *Measures of central tendency and range for player variables*
(N = 266)

Variables	Mean	SD	Median	Minimum	Maximum
Measurement occasions	34.61	37.23	22.00	10.00	246.00
Age (years)	53.08	16.33	55.55	18.32	85.85
Total playing days	157.08	140.54	127.00	1.00	872.00
Days per week	1.33	1.05	1.11	0.01	7.00
Total net loss ($)	884.33	14,406.02	3856.00	−258.00	107,989.00
Net loss per day ($)	54.80	63.72	31.59	−64.50	403.74
Total stroke	140,097.60	175,192.51	175,192.51	116.00	1,538,394.00
Stroke per day	842.91	526.54	720.24	14.50	2784.14

(NSW) have for many years, like casinos internationally, provided members with a personal card that, when entered in the machine as they start to play, records all plays and is used as a basis for promotions that reward high-spending players. The assistance of a machine manufacturer and a club enabled the reprogramming of the system to download individual player information (history/total plays, age and sex), all machines played, all plays by stake size, and net loss per occasion of play for each day's play.

The club operated 197 poker machines 7 days a week and held a membership base of about 16,000 adults. Restricting player sessions to net loss sessions, and a minimum of 10 recorded sessions per individual, a data collection period of 2 months gave 533 (53% women) players who played 18,077 occasions on 177 machines. Multilevel modelling was the preferred statistical procedure, giving a more accurate method of dealing with repeated measures (Goldstein, 1995). The statistical package MLn was selected, based on the review findings of Kreft et al. (1994).

The player descriptions at Table 3.2 above demonstrate that these regular players are indeed an "at-risk" group: net loss on any 1 day averaging $54, but ranging as high as $400. Total losses during membership ranged as high as $107,000.

The results for the variable stake size, for both samples/analyses, confirmed that machine denomination was able to explain just over 30% of the variance in stake size in both sets of data. In other words, as players moved from machine to machine, their stake size was influenced by the denomination of the machine. The maximum pay-lines variable weakly predicted player behaviour, accounting for less than 5% of the variance in both data sets. The results failed to support the hypothesis that the maximum bet influenced player behaviour.

The expectation that there would be variability between individuals in the effect size of either significant machine structural characteristic was confirmed, but this variation was not consistently accounted for by the predicted variable of the player's recorded total gaming experience. The analysis of player session loss confirmed only very weak relationships with structural characteristics and no confirmation of the impact of an individual's playing history. Thus, from the results of Study I, it could be concluded that the relationship between machine age and the presence of a bill acceptor and machine profitability was due to these machine characteristics attracting either a greater number of players, or players who spent more, rather than influencing the expenditure of individual players during a playing session.

In discussing the results, Haw noted that this was the first time that computer tracking, and machine-recorded data, had been subjected to inferential statistical analysis. Despite the gains in reliability in recording actual gaming behaviour in a venue, he noted that the record of a player's gaming history was limited to the individual's play in the club studied, and that it did not measure lifetime experiences. In addition, the data only recorded whether a machine was fitted with a bill acceptor, not whether a particular player had used it during their play on that machine.

Haw, never prone to theoretical speculation, reflected on several years immersed in the reality of the minutiae of EGMs:

"A major problem with operant conditioning explanations is the reported result for the denomination variable. Explaining the effect that denomination has on stake size with the 'size of reinforcement' principle, conflicts with the null result for the maximum bet multiplication variable. If increases in the size of reinforcement adequately explain the relationship between denomination and stake size, then the question must be asked why this principle did not apply to the maximum bet variable. . . . From the results for stake size, it was revealed that machine denomination was able to account for equal amounts of variance at both the occasion level and the player's level. However, the maximum pay-line variable was clearly accounting for variance at the occasion level. This implies that the denomination of a machine is also a player level variable (like age or gender or history of play). In other words, players may be defined by the denomination of the machines they play. This interpretation is similar to Griffiths' (1991b) observation of fruit machines in amusement arcades, where machines of different denominations appealed to different players based on gender and age.

If denomination is conceptualized both as a machine and a player variable, the descriptive and theoretical interpretation of the above results are altered. It also challenges the interpretation that Study I results were due to individual changes in stake size. It would appear that a machine's average stake size is due to a combination of attracting players (based on denomination) and also its ability to influence individual player's stake size (based on Pay-lines). The challenge that conceptualizing denomination as a player variable holds for contingency-based explanations of other variables, is that it suggests sensitivity to the response cost. That is, players may be controlling the size of the response cost via control of the denomination variable, rather than accepting the R-Sr contingency of denomination-wins. Therefore, explanations that encompass the response cost phenomenon may offer a more suitable explanation of the results.

The simple contingency principle of operant conditioning does not consider a schedule where both reinforcing and punishing stimuli are associated with the same response. It also fails to predict differential response effects for the frequency and size of reinforcement. Both these phenomena have been the domains of choice theories such as ecological learning and matching law (Chance, 1994; Davey, 1989; Lieberman, 1993). These theories utilize mathematical equations, which were considered inadequate explanations of poker machine play due to the negative or subtractive consequence of Type II punishment (measured in terms of size and frequency). In poker machine play, there exist a greater number of punished trials than reinforced, and under choice explanations, the gambling behaviour is itself an anomaly.

It was previously argued that poker machine play provided the opportunity to obtain a large reinforcer immediately at a relatively small response cost and, in combination with the ratio schedule of reinforcement, fostered a condition that promoted continuous risk-prone behaviour (Davey, 1989; Mazur, 1998). This may explain the appeal of games of chance, and therefore the control of machine denomination exhibited by players may be the means of controlling the response cost. Control of the frequency of response cost can only be governed by the number of pay-lines played and therefore the optimization problem facing the poker machine player may need to be conceptualized as one of minimizing response cost in the risk-prone behaviour, and not one of maximizing reinforcement. This is conducive with the findings of other studies suggesting that players are aware that a loss will be incurred and adopt a strategy to maximize playing time (Walker, 1992b)." (Haw, 2000, pp. 246–247)

. . . "**The only theoretical conclusion that can be drawn from the above results is that the operant conditioning predictions were not supported**. The machine variable with an established R-Sr contingency, in terms of reinforcement frequency (maximum pay-lines) was related to average stake size, but the machine variable with an established R-Sr contingency, in terms of reinforcement size (maximum bet), was not related to average stake size. The result for the machine denomination variable suggests that size of reinforcement is important, but . . . it would appear to both influence a player's stake size and be utilized by players to control stake size. **This introduces the notion of response cost, which is problematic for learning explanations**." (Haw, 2000, p. 249 emphasis added)

Haw's work was based on a thorough knowledge of the machines and players that he was studying; the data he used as the basis for his analyses was ecologically valid. This approach, linked with a greater depth of psychologically relevant measures at the level of the individual in a multilevel analysis, provides a unique methodology for the future study of gambling behaviour. The large proportion of unexplained variance in Haw's analyses at both the machine and the individual level confirms there is scope for the inclusion of other variables.

The failure to find support for operant derived hypotheses about quite fundamental themes such as size of reinforcement, confirms that earlier speculations about structural effects (e.g. Griffiths, 1993b) and proposals to change structural characteristics to protect problem players are unlikely to be supported by ecologically valid empirical data. This anticipates the discussion in Chapter 6 of the recent studies completed in Canada and Australia that examined changes to machine structural characteristics with a view to retaining their attraction to ordinary players, but removing the "addictive" process that impacted on problem players.

The results for the Scale of Gambling Choices (SGC) presented in the previous chapter confirmed how common was the experience of some level of impaired control amongst regular players such as those studied by Haw. In attempting to link his results to self-control it would be tempting, but possibly quite incorrect, to speculate that the more that an individual player's pattern of staking was accounted for by structural characteristics, the more the player might report impaired control. The challenge to this is that the regular players who comprised Haw's sample typically played 10 different machines during a session. This is confirmed by Walker (2004) for data derived in a similar way from player tracking data, and led him to comment on how the picture of a player moving around the venue "selecting" machines to play differed from the common assumption that problem players were engrossed in continuous play.

The Nature of Reinforcement in Gambling

The assumption underlying Skinner's (1953) original claim regarding the role of the slot machine in generating pathological involvement in gambling was that the intermittent reinforcement of a cash payout was the secondary reinforcer. Walker (1992b) undermines this, pointing out that most gambling responses are followed by a cost or loss that could be considered aversive. Even if cash won *is* a contributor to learning, taken alone it would be unlikely to contribute to a type of learning that in both regular and problem gambling is seen to be habitual and resistant to extinction. Strength of learning is mediated by:

1. R-Sr contiguity, with shorter delays between staking/bet placement and its consequent "reward", but R-Sr contiguity (for cash) for example may vary

from 5 s in EGM play to several minutes in horse race betting, and even longer if there is an inquiry into a result.
2. Individual differences in prior learning, that is experience of the gambling form.
3. VR schedules (Chance, 1994), except during initial shaping of behaviour when continuous reinforcement is effective.

The intermittent nature of cash reinforcement has also been problematic in accounting for initial stages of learning to regularly consume a particular form of continuous gambling such as off-course betting, EGM play or casino table games. The initial stages of this learning have not been the focus of research, but observations and comparisons between infrequent and regular gamblers suggest that behavioural-shaping results in the more stereotypic gambling responses of regular players; effective shaping requires continuous reinforcement.

An early article by Dickerson (1979) reported the survey and direct observation results of the betting behaviour of regular gamblers in off-course venues in Birmingham (UK). Commenting on the strong observed relationship between the time of bet placement in the few moments before the "off" (the start of the broadcast race when no more bets on that race are accepted), Dickerson speculated that if this stereotypic pattern were the result of shaping (infrequent bettors placed bets much earlier in the temporal sequence of events), then in terms of the timing/contiguity of reinforcement, what may be occurring just after bet placement is reinforcing, increasingly so when placed immediately prior to the "off"? Certainly winning is far removed in terms of timing.

It can be argued that for all forms of gambling the universe changes once a stake has been placed: Oldman (1978) called it "hope" while working as a casino croupier/sociological observer in Aberdeen (Scotland) and provocatively wrote of parallels between his sightings of winning compulsive gamblers and the Yeti. The hope for a win existed despite the expectation of losing. Whether one accepts the term "hope" or not, the reality of the change in a gambler's universe is underpinned by an indisputable and perhaps remorseless logic. For example, Oldman observed a person, due to appear in court the next day over gambling debts, gambling with the last of his available cash. On purely logical grounds such behaviour could, he argued, be understood; not to gamble ensured that his debts would remain; to gamble gave the possibility of debt reduction or elimination as well as the possibility of a small (relative) increase in his debts.

Reinforcement that maintains regular gambling may be the cognitive–emotional experience, its positive valence and intensity, that is associated with what Oldman called hope and which occurs immediately after the stake is placed. In continuous forms of gambling, the relatively slower paced sequences of reinforcement in, for example, off-course betting, may be as effective as for the faster cycles of EGM play and casino table games because of the greater strength of the experienced emotion arising from the race commentary immediately following bet placement. The effectiveness of this reinforcement for the regular gambler may be undermined if staking is made well before the "off", not just by the loss of contiguity but also because time remains for new information to be processed as odds continue to change, anxiety that the "wrong" horse has been backed and even further staking on other runners in the same race. Such repeated betting on the same race have been observed (e.g. Newman, 1972).

Statistically unusual outcomes such as big wins, sequences of repeated losses or wins as well as "near-misses", may generate particularly strong and reinforcing emotional experiences in all forms of continuous gambling. In EGM play the positive emotional experience may be *sustained* by continuing to play rather than each stake or purchase of a game resulting in a subjectively detectable emotional change. It can be speculated that expectations will play a significant role both for "session start" and "session stop". With regard to starting a session, where the expectation of positive emotional experience and hope of winning is more notable for regular players if they have current dysphoric mood, a form of the decision theory model subjective expected emotion (SEE) (Mellers et al., 1999) may be a relevant conceptual model. In contrast, "session end" may be better accounted for in terms of Regret Theory (Baron, 1994) or avoidance of the strong negative emotional experience that the player expects to occur once gambling ceases. Thus regular players during the latter stages of a long session may describe continuing to play despite the lack of any positive enjoyment, but merely to prevent the enormous regret associated with another player winning "their" money (O'Connor & Dickerson, 1997).

Recent research linking expectations of winning money with measurable physiological markers such as cortical responses (Breiter et al., 2001) and heart rate increases (Ladouceur et al., 2003) provides support for these speculations (reviewed in greater detail below).

Prior Mood and Emotion while Gambling

There is a growing body of observational, clinical and survey research that has implicated dysphoric mood in excessive gambling. Low mood prior to the commencement of a session on EGMs has been linked to persistence when losing (Corless & Dickerson, 1989; Dickerson et al., 1991), and this relationship has also been found in British fruit-machine players (Griffiths, 1995b). Feelings of frustration and disappointment have been associated with an increased likelihood of beginning a session amongst EGM players with high impaired control (Corless & Dickerson, 1989).

In community surveys of regular gamblers, depression and anxiety were nominated as reasons for starting sessions (Dickerson et al., 1996b). Twenty-eight per cent of "problem EGM players" played to forget their troubles and worries compared to just 4% of regular (but non-problematic) players (Schellinck & Schrans, 1998). Dysphoric mood was found to be related to high South Oaks Gambling Screen (SOGS) scores in both male and female EGM players in a community sample (Ohtsuka et al., 1997).

Depression and, to a lesser extent, anxiety are common at presentation in clinical samples of gamblers (Ramirez et al., 1983; McCormick et al., 1984; Ciarrocchi, 1987; Battersby & Tolchard, 1996; Specker et al., 1996; Stinchfield & Winters, 1996), and treatment outcome research has implicated low mood in relapse (Blaszczynski et al., 1991a, b). In a study comparing "pathological gamblers" with heroin "addicts" and controls on the Eysenck Personality Questionnaire, it was concluded that the "similarities between pathological gamblers and substance addicts may reflect a general factor of affective disturbance" (Blaszczynski et al., 1985, p. 315). However, the issue of whether depression precedes and contributes to the development of excessive gambling, or is a consequence of over-involvement, awaits clarification from longitudinal research (Walker, 1992b).

Related to mood states, emotional arousal has featured prominently in explanations of persistent gambling (Goffman, 1969; Anderson & Brown, 1984; Leary & Dickerson, 1985; Brown, 1986, 1987; Dickerson & Adcock, 1987; Moodie & Finnigan, 2005). Dickerson and Adcock (1987), on the basis of subjective report and physiological measures that showed high-frequency gamblers to be more aroused, proposed a model to integrate mood and cognition. It was suggested that those with low mood would show greater persistence when losing as a consequence of reduced habituation to arousal. It was argued that cognitive distortion occurs with higher arousal levels, so that the illusion of control is more pronounced. However, further research by Dickerson et al. (1991) led to a conclusion that low mood might be more significant than arousal in persistent EGM play, though it is recognised that this finding may not generalise to other forms of gambling (Dickerson, 1991).

Horse-race gamblers have reported experiencing much excitement (Dickerson, 1979; Lesieur, 1984; Rosecrance, 1986; Orford et al., 1996), and when their heart rates were monitored, significant increases were demonstrated (Coventry & Brown, 1993; Coventry & Norman, 1997). Likewise, heart rates in casino gamblers have been found to increase substantially, with increases of up to 53 beats/min when recorded during play in a casino (Anderson & Brown, 1984). Heavily involved fruit-machine players reported more excitement than their less involved counterparts (Griffiths, 1991b). This is confirmed for regular EGM players by subjective reports combined with physiological measures (Leary & Dickerson, 1985; Moodie & Finnigan, 2005). Increased arousal levels were measured in "problem gamblers" (horse-race gamblers and EGM players) when just watching a video of a horse race or an EGM being played, and imagining their own participation (Sharpe et al., 1995).

In a comparison of EGM players and horse-race gamblers, EGM players reported being more anxious and were keen to avoid arousal, whereas the horse-race gamblers preferred heightened arousal (Cocco et al., 1995). However, in other research, female fruit-machine players' heart rates were elevated when they experienced a win or anticipated a win (Coventry & Hudson, 2001), and Canadian EGM regular players have reported pounding hearts, butterflies in the stomach and sweaty hands or body during play (Schellinck & Schrans, 1998).

Recent Canadian studies have clarified some of the outstanding issues concerning the subjective and physiological measures of arousal in gaming machine play. Diskin and colleagues (Diskin & Hodgins, 2003; Diskin et al., 2003) confirmed that neither subjective ratings of excitement and tension, nor heart rate and skin conductance measures during gaming in a laboratory and in a venue, revealed differences between gamblers grouped according to their scores above or below 5 on the SOGS (Lesieur & Blume, 1987). This may be indicative of the value of separating level of involvement in gambling from impaired self-control rather than using a heterogeneous measure of pathological gambling.

Ladouceur and colleagues in Quebec used heart rate during gaming machine play and retrospective subjective reports of excitement to evaluate the independent variable of expectations of winning (Ladouceur et al., 2003). The study was completed in a university laboratory setting, but recruited current infrequent and monthly players by advertisement and used a current video lottery terminal (VLT) machine, an eight-line fruit game called "Swinging Bells". After playing 50 games under the known return rate of 92%, participants were advised that they could, in the next 50 games, win at a return rate of 200% (the experimental group up to $40 and the other group credits only). During the rest period of 1 min that followed this information, the experimental group showed significantly higher heart rate, which was sustained while gaming, and subsequently higher subjective ratings of excitement. Although the authors discussed the results in terms of high and low expectations, this conclusion was not warranted as the control group were not actually gambling. The study does confirm existing literature (Breiter et al., 2001) that expectations of winning **are** important in generating a significant change in the emotions experienced by gamblers. It indicates that in studies such as Dickerson et al. (1992), where no change in heart rate was found for regular players from baseline to first plays on a gaming machine, that it was the method that was the problem: the baseline measures were taken in the venue immediately prior to play when expectations might well have already raised the players pulse rate.

A second concern about the Ladouceur study is the failure to distinguish between regular and infrequent players. As we argued earlier, there is a variety of supporting evidence that regular players of continuous forms are significantly more vulnerable to the harmful impacts of gambling than infrequent players and that this is in some way a function of their greater conditioning or learning that has resulted in more stereotypic or habitual gambling behaviours. If the excitement generated by expectations of winning are an important contributor to maintaining play, and perhaps to the process of eroding self-control, then comparisons of infrequent and regular players should show different patterns of excitement, as found in Hills et al. (2001).

In critiquing the gambling literature on mood and emotion, Hills et al. (2001) emphasised the confounding of the two primary dimensions of emotion, namely affective valence (pleasant to unpleasant) and arousal (Diener, 1999; Russell & Barrett, 1999; Watson et al., 1999). The latter is only rewarding when positively valenced and typical physiological measures of arousal such as heart rate and skin conductance are unable to reliably distinguish valence. Depressed mood within this framework is more appropriately considered as negatively valenced low arousal. In contrast, relaxation is positively valued low arousal and may therefore be rewarding. Support for this in regular gamblers (VLT players), with and without problems, is to be found in Schrans et al. (2000). These authors reported that almost a quarter of regular players who were still experiencing problems of control cited relaxation, and the chance to calm down and escape from their problems as motivation to gamble.

The only experimental study of the impact of induced prior mood on gambling behaviour and highlights both the gains and the costs of the laboratory study of gambling (Hills et al., 2001). Using a computerised card game (Breen & Zuckerman, 1999), male students who were regular and infrequent EGM players were recruited and randomly allocated to one of three prior mood inductions: elated, depressed and neutral mood. Mood was monitored before, during and after gaming, and their duration of play while losing was recorded. The results showed that the depressed infrequent players persisted less than the neutral or elated infrequent players, an effect not shown by the regulars who appeared motivated to gamble regardless of their prior mood or their mounting losses. Rather than prior depressed mood acting to increase persistent play, it appeared that regular players had "lost" the inhibition shown by the depressed infrequent players. In addition, the tracking results showed that regular players showed greater increases in positive mood during play than infrequent players and also, having lost, showed the largest fall in positive mood after play. These results for the regular players were interpreted in terms of the potential for mood repair provided by a session of gambling, and that the subsequent depressed mood should the player lose would not be a factor inhibiting future sessions.

The results from this laboratory study, albeit well designed and involving actual risking of cash, illustrate the need to check such results with evidence from the real world of gambling. The inhibitory effect of depressed mood on infrequent players was found by the survey study of Corless & Dickerson (1989), but the lack of support for the expected association between prior depressed mood and impaired control over session spend (e.g. Dickerson & Adcock, 1987; Griffiths, 1995a) highlights the frailty of assuming that persistence in the laboratory while losing is an analogue of impaired control.

There are two strands to theory and investigation of arousal at the biochemical level in relation to excessive behaviours, both of which are speculative at this time. One is the notion that excessive behaviours are mediated by greater or lesser levels of neurotransmitters (perhaps dopamine) than found in the general population (e.g. Jacobs, 1987). It is hypothesised that this process may occur as a secondary phenomenon when some other abnormal state (e.g. depression or anxiety, impulsivity) is involved in dysfunction of neurochemistry (Blaszczynski & Nower, 2002). An attempt at self-medication may occur via the mood enhancing or modulating effects of, for example, gambling. Anderson & Brown (1984) applied reversal theory to excessive gambling, hypothesising that both low arousal (relief from boredom and achieving relaxation) and high arousal (relief from anxiety and achieving excitement) can, in the same individual, be implicated in motives for starting to gamble and continuing to gamble.

The second strand of biochemical theorising is that gambling itself may alter arousal levels, prompting changes in neurochemistry which endure beyond gambling sessions. It is conceivable that a degree of neuroadaptation (akin to tolerance in drug use) occurs in whichever greater levels of gambling are required for the individual to achieve homoeostatic functioning. Neuroadaptation can result in withdrawal symptoms, markedly so for some drugs, and possibly when there is an abrupt cessation of regular, heavy levels of gambling (Wray & Dickerson, 1981; Rosenthal & Lesieur, 1992; Bergh & Kulhorn, 1994).

Personality

There is a large literature on personality characteristics and excessive gambling, but very little specifically in relation to impaired control. The general area will, therefore, be only briefly outlined. The whole area is characterised by inconsistent and inconclusive findings (Murray, 1993; Dickerson & Baron, 2000).

Psychoanalytic speculation has stressed developmental crises in the family of origin that result in low self-esteem in childhood. Gambling is thought to be a means to escape (disassociate from) negative feelings and to raise self-esteem through being a winner (Lesieur, 1984; Jacobs, 1987; see Walker, 1992b, for a review). Under these conditions, losing is thought to be an extremely aversive state, with chasing an attempt not only to win back losses, but also to restore fragile self-esteem (Lesieur, 1984). The most popularised psychoanalytic notion of excessive gamblers is that they subconsciously wish to lose in order to punish themselves (Bergler, 1957). There is no evidence as yet supporting psychoanalytic theorising, and it is difficult to see how it could be obtained given the hypothesised role of the subconscious.

The personality variables that have received the most attention in excessive gamblers are sensation-seeking, extraversion and locus-of-control (Walker, 1992b). The findings are inconsistent (possibly reflecting the fact that very different subgroups have been recruited to studies), with sensation-seeking and extraversion found to be at both lower and higher levels in excessive gamblers than in the general population and in low-frequency gamblers (Walker, 1992b; Dickerson & Baron, 2000). Locus-of-control is usually more external in excessive gamblers, but in a number of studies there were no differences to controls (Walker, 1992b). Inconsistent results such as these led Murray (1993) to conclude that "pathological gamblers vary tremendously on many dimensions" (p. 793).

However, within some subpopulations of gamblers, certain personality characteristics are commonly found. In a sample of Gamblers Anonymous (GA) members and gamblers receiving psychiatric inpatient treatment, elevated impulsivity scores have been detected (Blaszczynski et al.,1997). This is also the case for excessive alcohol and other drug use; such findings seem to be the result of tapping a subpopulation of males (previously often labelled antisocial personality disorder) who experience multiple life difficulties (reviewed by Knapp & Lech, 1987; McCown, 1988). This interpretation is supported by factor analysis in which an "impulsive antisocial factor was found to be associated with gambling behaviour and indices of poor psychosocial functioning" (Steel & Blaszczynski, 1996, p. 3). In a laboratory-based analogue of gambling,

Zuckerman's impulsivity factor (Zuckerman-Kuhlman Personality Question-naire, Zuckerman et al., 1993) predicted higher-average bets, but *not* persistence when losing, leading Breen & Zuckerman (1999) to conclude that impulsive-ness may have "more to do with the willingness to participate in gambling gen-erally, or to begin a new session of gambling" (p. 54). Impulsivity in 12–14-year olds of low socio-economic status was found to predict excessive gambling later in their teens (Vitaro et al., 1999).

The American Psychiatric Association (1994) has located pathological gam-bling within the diagnostic category "disorders of impulse control" in the *Diagnostic and Statistical Manual of Mental Disorders, 4th edition* (DSM-IV). However, as Murray (1993) discussed, impulse control disorders are a diag-nostic group that is not well understood, and indeed there is far from universal agreement that such a classification has validity or utility. It is very problematic with regard to gambling, as it implies "irresistible impulses", yet much plan-ning can be involved when raising finances to further the chase (Lesieur, 1984). Indeed, Lesieur's impression was that his respondents had to "learn the trade" of financing "the chase".

Though more than a decade has passed since their comprehensive review, Knapp and Lech's (1987) conclusion that the "utility and values of such studies remain doubtful" still seems valid, and they cautioned against "characterizing the pathological gambler as possessing a particular personality type" (p. 33). If progress is to be made in this area, it seems necessary to investigate personal-ity within ecologically valid gambling settings (Dickerson, 1991), and to relate it to specific, definable, aspects of excessive gambling.

Alcohol

Harm to the individual and the family that may extend into the community is associated with the juxtaposition of two favourite leisure activities in most "western" nations, gambling and the consumption of alcohol. As is commonly the case worldwide, both are licensed and made available in the same venue such as a social club, hotel, bar or casino. Underpinning this legalised avail-ability is the generally accepted gambling policy objective that gambling, espe-cially gaming machines, should be available in a context where there is on offer a range of leisure activities, where the customer has a choice of leisure and entertainment activities. Accumulating evidence of the ways in which drinking alcohol and gambling may interact to cause a complex mix of both gambling- and alcohol-related problems challenges this policy assumption.

Rates of Problem Gambling in Clinical Samples of Alcohol
and Substance Abuse

Studies that report rates of pathological gambling in substance abusing patients in the USA have been generally consistent in their findings. Results of a study by McCormick (1993) revealed that of the 2171 substance abusers in treatment, 9.9% that abused alcohol scored 5 or more on the SOGS (Lesieur & Blume, 1987). Ciarrocchi's (1987), study of 467 substance (including alcohol) abusing patients found 10.7% scoring 5 or more on SOGS. Lejoyeux et al. (1999) found 8.9% of alcohol abusers meeting the criteria for problem gambling in a sample of patients receiving treatment for an impulse control disorder. Lesieur et al. (1986) found 5% of the 458 patients being treated for alcohol problems at the South Oaks Hospital scored 5 or more on SOGS. In addition, Lesieur et al. (1986) found that 34% of their patients being treated for alcohol and drugs reported gambling while drinking or using drugs "some of the time", while 5% reported "most" or "all of the time", thereby shedding some light on the process of interaction between the two behaviours.

Higher rates of co-morbid substance abuse and problem gambling have been found in other studies. For example, Daghestani et al. (1996) found a rate of 33% of problem gamblers (i.e. scoring 5 or more on the SOGS) in a sample of 276 substance abusers. In a study of 462 patients in methadone treatment programs in New York (Spunt et al., 1998), 30% were problem gamblers scoring 5 or more on SOGS, and 47% of the sample used alcohol just prior to or during gambling. The results indicated further that alcohol was more likely to be consumed while gambling than cocaine (23%), marijuana (17%) or other drugs (10%). A study examining rates of pathological gambling amongst Native Americans and Caucasian patients in treatment for alcohol dependence ($N = 85$) found 22% Native Americans (versus 7% in Caucasians) had co-morbid gambling problems (Elia & Jacobs, 1993).

Rates of Alcohol and Substance Abuse in Clinical Samples
of Problem Gamblers

A small number of studies in the US on problem gamblers in treatment reveal similarly high rates of co-morbid substance abuse. For instance, Ramirez et al. (1983) found 39% of pathological gamblers undergoing treatment at the Veteran Administration Medical Centre met the criteria for alcohol misuse or drug misuse in the last year, and 47% of the sample met the criteria at some point in their life. Ciarrocchi and Richardson (1989) found 34% of 186 patients admitted to a private psychiatric hospital for problem gambling had co-morbid alcohol problems. Templer et al. (1993) found problem gambling to be significantly correlated with scores on the MacAndrews Alcoholism Scale. Linden et al. (1986) reported 52% alcohol abuse rate with GA members. Similarly, Lesieur and Blume (1991) found that 52% of 50 women problem gamblers attending GA had abused alcohol and/or drugs at some time in their lives.

More recently in Australia, the Productivity Commission's (1999) national inquiry into the economic, individual and social impacts of gambling in Australia revealed that about one in five severe problem gamblers attending problem gambling services were reported to be suffering from co-morbid alcoholism or other chemical dependencies.

There are of course many problems associated with the selective and therefore possibly unrepresentative nature of clinical samples (e.g. for problem gambling, Volberg & Steadman, 1988) and it is fortunate that the literature now includes several co-morbidity estimates derived from samples of the general population.

Non-Clinical Samples with Problem Drinking/Problem Gambling Co-morbidity

Most recent studies on non-clinical co-morbid samples have come from Australia, Canada, New Zealand and the USA, and include both survey-based and experimental designs. The results indicate high rates of co-morbid problem drinking/problem gambling in non-clinical samples.

Smart and Ferris (1996) conducted a study, which examined the relationship between alcohol, drugs and gambling in Ontario, Canada. Using a telephone survey approach, 2016 randomly selected Ontario adults participated and results indicated problem gambling was significantly related to problem drinking, smoking and other drug use. The most significant predictors of problem gambling were expenditure on gambling, alcohol dependence and age.

In the USA, a study examining the association between problem gambling and other psychiatric disorders using data from the St Louis epidemiological catchment area indicated that, of the 161 individuals assessed to be problem gamblers, 44% met the criteria for alcohol dependence. Among the problem gamblers with alcohol problems, gambling problems occurred within 2 years of the onset of alcoholism in 65% of cases (Cunningham-Williams et al., 1998).

In a 7-year follow-up study on frequent and problem gambling in New Zealand, Abbott et al. (1999) found that 40% lifetime probable pathological gamblers (SOGS) experienced alcohol-related problems in 1991, and 54% of those people continued to experience alcohol-related problems in 1999.

College samples in the USA also reveal high rates of concurrent drinking and gambling problems. For example, Lesieur et al. (1991), found in a sample of 1771 university students that 5.5% were problem gamblers, with SOGS scores correlating significantly with measures of alcohol abuse. In a study examining overlapping addictions in college men and women, Greenberg et al. (1999) reported that men scored higher than women did on addictions to alcohol, cigarettes, gambling, television and the Internet. Women scored higher on caffeine and chocolate. Barnes et al. (1999), in a study exploring the predictors of gambling and alcohol behaviour among youth in New York, found that impulsivity, "moral disengagement" and delinquency predicted alcohol consumption and gambling. Very similar trends were found in a large study of children and adolescents in Australia (DHS, 1999). Also in Australia, a research team evaluated the social and economic impact of regular gambling in NSW by a random door-knock household survey (Dickerson et al., 1998). Results showed that almost 40% of men and 15% of women at risk of gambling problems (i.e. SOGS score of 5 or more) associated with regular consumption of continuous forms of gambling (e.g. EGM, casino, racing and cards) scored 8 or more on the Alcohol Use Disorders Identification Test (AUDIT), that is at least into the hazardous drinking category. This compared to less than 5% of women and approximately 20% of men at risk of problems associated with discontinuous forms of gambling (e.g. Lotto, Oz lotto, Powerball and the Lottery) scored 8 or more on the AUDIT.

The most recent study (Dickerson et al., 2001) sampled three high-risk populations within a single jurisdiction, regular EGM players recruited in venues, individuals attending treatment for either alcohol or gambling problems (or both), and a media-recruited sample of self-identified problem gamblers or problem drinkers not currently attending treatment and who had not attended for treatment in the last 12 months. The latter two groups were predominantly male and for alcohol problems in treatment or not in treatment the co-morbidity rates (using scores of 5 and more on the SOGS, and 8 and more on the AUDIT) were 38% and 50%, respectively. The co-morbidity of alcohol problems in the matching problem gambler groups was higher, 48% and 58%, respectively. The results from the sample of 154 regular EGM players, of whom 46% were women, showed that 20% were problem gamblers, 13% were problem drinkers and 20% satisfied both criteria, that is 46% had neither gambling or alcohol problems. The co-morbidity rates for women were somewhat lower than for men and there was a predominance of the age group 20–29 years in the co-morbid group. The 20% co-morbidity for regular EGM players was half the rate found in the earlier random-based population survey (Dickerson et al., 1998). This may in part be because of the sampling method used, but the latter sample also included problem gamblers who preferred other forms such as off-course betting and casino gaming that may be associated with higher levels of risk of excessive alcohol consumption.

Thus the evidence suggests that the co-morbidity estimates from clinical samples fall within the range found in general population studies depending on the jurisdiction and probably the types of gambling products available. Youth studies suggest that there may be an early developmental pattern associated with the uptake of both gambling and drinking alcohol to levels considered harmful (DHS, 2000) and Maddern (2004) in a qualitative study of youth regular gamblers recorded that it was the self-regulated gamblers who were more aware of the way in which drinking alcohol impaired their ability to maintain self-control over time and money expenditure. She speculated that for those who were not self-regulated their experience of gambling was so beset with problems and emotions of guilt and frustration that they were less likely to detect and comment upon the impact of alcohol on their gambling decisions.

The interaction of the two leisure behaviours of gambling and drinking has rarely been studied but it would be anticipated that consumption of alcohol, notoriously associated with impaired decision-making and increased risk-taking behaviours (Chesher & Greeley, 1989), will have a cogent impact on gambling choices. A gambler's choice to resist urges to either start or stop gambling and to limit expenditure may be seriously affected under the influence of alcohol. Indeed the relationship may be much more complex than simply alcohol disinhibiting subjective control of gambling (Blaszczynski & McConaghy, 1988). The relationship may well be cyclical, with alcohol leading to problematic gambling, and/or gambling losses precipitating alcohol misuse.

There are just two studies examining how the processes of drinking alcohol and gambling may interact to erode subjective control over these leisure behaviours.

The first Baron and Dickerson (1999) recruited men and women players as they sat at a card machine beginning a session of play (study preceded the NSW introduction of poker machines to hotels and bars). The results showed that one in eight gamblers reported difficulty resisting urges to gamble (and actually were playing EGMs when interviewed) after consuming on average at least two standard alcoholic drinks while in the gaming venue (i.e. a bar/hotel), despite having made an earlier determination not to gamble that day.

A second study by Kyngdon and Dickerson (1999) examined the interaction of alcohol and gambling in an experimental setting. Male participants ($N = 40$, mean age $= 20.7$ years) were recruited who regularly both drank alcohol and played gaming machines. (The pre-existing habits of drinking at least three standard alcoholic drinks in a session and regular EGM play was an ethical requirement before the study could proceed.) They were assigned randomly to one of two groups. In the experimental group they drank three alcoholic drinks and in the control three placebo drinks while completing a personality inventory (NEO; Costa & McCrae, 1992a) before gambling on a simulated EGM (Breen & Zuckerman, 1999). Results revealed that those in the alcohol group played twice as many trials as those in the placebo group, with significantly more players losing all of their original cash staked (50% versus 15% in the placebo group). Although the dependent variable of persistence while losing may be challenged as an acceptable experimental equivalent of impaired control, session duration is typically the best predictor of impaired control (e.g. Corless & Dickerson 1989; Baron & Dickerson, 1999). The sample of players had a mean score on the SGC (mean = 42.68) very similar to other samples of men and women regular players recruited in venues. The personality results, although not the focus of the study, produced a glimpse of the complexity of the interactions that may contribute to self-control of gambling behaviour: the placebo group showed a significant and positive relationship between depressed mood and persistence but it was noted that the absence of the same relationship in the experimental group may have been because the alcohol consumption lifted their mood, altering their responses to the depression items. To examine the predictiveness of depression, extraversion and excitement-seeking scores on the number of game trials played by participants administered the placebo, a stepwise multiple regression analysis was conducted; excitement-seeking emerged as the only significant predictor of the number of trials played, accounting for 27% of the variance. Higher scores on excitement-seeking predicted *less* persistence, fewer trails before stopping gaming, a result entirely compatible with the lower than average mean scores on the Sensation-Seeking Scale found for regular off-course gamblers recruited in venues (Dickerson et al., 1987). On the face of it EGM play is likely to be much less "exciting" than off-course betting and this is supported by the greater difficulty in measuring any significant physiological changes indicative of excitement or arousal in players while gaming in venues rather than in laboratories (Leary & Dickerson, 1985; Dickerson et al., 1991, 1992).

The really interesting finding by Kyngdon and Dickerson (1999) was that the alcohol group showed none of the significant personality relationships. It can be speculated that perhaps young males who are high on personality variables that are associated with a low interest in gambling on EGMs may visit a bar or hotel, perhaps even having determined not to gamble that night (Baron &

Dickerson, 1999), consume a social, "responsible" level of alcohol, and then find the prospect of gambling an attractive option. This suggests that the empirical associations between problem gambling and personality variables such as impulsivity (e.g. Steel & Blaszczynski, 1996) that are included in the pathways model may give very little insight into the underlying complexity of the psychological processes that lead to harmful levels of gambling.

Interview data from a study of video lottery players in Nova Scotia Schellinck and Schrans (1998) showing that although some players drank more while playing a similar proportion drank less is an important reminder that it should not be assumed on the basis of a few studies that the marketing of alcohol and gambling at the same venue is necessarily harmful. The complex interrelationship between the two behaviours reinforces, Korn et al.'s (2003) argument that gambling impacts should be interpreted within the public health domain. From the evidence it is clear that the development of public health strategies concerning problem gambling and drinking need to be coordinated within the community rather than being primarily a treatment issue.

The Role of Cognitive Variables

There is a significant body of literature on cognitive distortions of probability, particularly misinterpretations of randomness involved in gambling (reviewed in Griffiths, 1990, 1996; Walker, 1992b; Sharpe & Tarrier, 1993; Ladouceur and Walker, 1996). A cognitive perspective on excessive gambling and impaired control "assumes that the utility of gambles is sometimes misperceived ... and focuses on the frequent or regular gambler and the explanation for his or her persistence with gambling despite losses" (Ladouceur & Walker, 1996, p. 93).

Perhaps the most notable erroneous belief is the "illusion of control" in which the gambler believes they can influence outcomes that are actually chance determined (Langer, 1975). In a series of studies, Langer demonstrated that when an element of skill is perceived to apply to a chance outcome, the illusion of control may be magnified. The conditions under which this occurred were those where subjects exercised choice, had familiarity with the task, had direct personal involvement, and perceived competitors as being less skilled. In relation to the choice variable, the illusion of control was so powerful that the subjects forfeited the right to exercise real control by refusing to accept better odds.

Lesieur (1984) noted that faith in a "system" (a set of calculations that the gambler believes will allow predictions to be made) is often associated with one particular aspect of impaired control, chasing. Superstitious behaviour, where ritualistic behaviour is engaged in to promote luck, is also considered an example of an illusion of control (Ladouceur & Walker, 1996). Cognitive theorists argue that chasing is more likely if an illusion of control is operating (Walker, 1992b) given the belief that persistence will be eventually rewarded.

Other common cognitive errors relating to probability include representative and availability bias. Representative bias occurs when inferences are made on limited sampling. The extremely common cognitive error in which it is believed that knowledge of past outcomes of a random nature allow prediction of future outcomes (the "gambler's fallacy") is the classic example of representative bias (Wagenaar, 1988). Availability bias refers to "reducing complex probabilistic judgements to simpler ones through the ease to which relevant instances can be brought to mind" (Corney & Cummings, 1985, p. 111).

Wagenaar (1988) summarised a total of 16 cognitive distortions that operate in the context of gambling, leading him to conclude that most gamblers do not understand randomness. Gamblers do not seem to abide by normative models of decision-making (strictly utilitarian pay-off), but this is hardly surprising as there is a long history of research indicating that humans, whether gambling or not, perform less than rationally, particularly under conditions of uncertainty (Janis & Mann, 1977). Some of these cognitive errors seem to be part of most gambling, whereas others (e.g. the illusion of control) seem to speak more directly to the conditions under which chasing may occur such as in off-course betting.

Subsequent to Langer's (1975) seminal research, it has been consistently demonstrated that erroneous perceptions when engaged in gambling tasks are the norm. Gaboury & Ladouceur (1989) pioneered the technique of having subjects verbalise their thoughts while playing, and a number of studies employing the "thinking aloud method" (notwithstanding concerns about the intrusiveness of this methodology) have consistently shown the presence of erroneous perceptions and beliefs (Ladouceur & Walker, 1996). Regular gamblers on fruit-machines are more prone to cognitive distortions than are non-regular players (Griffiths, 1990, 1994b). In some cases players might not express any faulty beliefs away from the "action", but succumb to erroneous perceptions during play (Dickerson, 1991). False beliefs whilst playing EGMs was recently found to be associated with greater risk taking (Delfabbro & Winefield, 2000).

Lesieur (1984) commented that chasing gamblers often believe they are better gamblers than the average gambler, so not only are they trying to recoup losses, but they are also attempting to recover their positive gambling-related self-identities and esteem. If faulty perceptions are coupled to "core beliefs" that one is knowledgeable and skilful, that one has the resources to be successful, and that persistence will be rewarded, then chasing (particularly the attempt to recoup losses by increasing the size of bets) is likely, according to Walker (1992b). Twenty-seven per cent of "problem EGM players" in a large random household survey felt they had the ability to influence the outcome, compared to 13% of frequent, but non-problematic, players (Schellinck & Schrans, 1998). Of the problem players, 64% admitted to regularly chasing their losses.

Another complexity is that over the course of a gambling career, the subjective value of stakes and pay-outs is likely to alter (Lesieur, 1984; Wagenaar, 1988). As the subjective value of stakes diminishes over time, the amount wagered increases. An increase in staking levels is considered to be a common feature of chasing, particularly when chasing behaviour is well established (Lesieur, 1984; Walker, 1992b). Corless & Dickerson (1989) found that EGM gamblers who showed more persistence when losing had notions of a "big win" that were twice those of high-frequency (but non-problem) and low-frequency gamblers. Additionally, their gambling expenditure was twice that of high-frequency gamblers, and more than 200 times that of low-frequency gamblers. Lesieur's (1984) sample of GA members had increased their wagers incrementally over the course of their gambling, as the values of their stakes subjectively diminished, and they often changed to betting strategies that provided the chance of bigger returns (e.g. backing a horse with longer odds). The behaviour of attempting to recover past losses by further gambling is consistent with anticipated wins having greater saliency, or value, than money already lost (Wagenaar, 1988). This was conceptualised by Lesieur (1984), on the basis of Devereux's thesis (1949, cited in the reference of Lesieur), that certain losses are more aversive than are potential losses contingent on future events.

Chasing has also been conceptualised as a process of being over-committed to a failing strategy (Lesieur, 1984). Rosecrance (1986) wrote of the persistence and commitment demonstrated by serious gamblers after they had suffered a heavy loss. In contrast, Lesieur (1984) and Custer (1984) believed that big wins early in the career of the "chaser" were more critical than losses, establishing a belief that further big wins are likely. It has been suggested by Walker (1992b) that the notion of "entrapment" may be of relevance here. Entrapment is "a decision-making process whereby individuals' escalate their commitment to a previously chosen, though failing, course of action in order to justify or 'make good on' prior investments" (Brockner & Rubin, 1985; cited in Walker, 1992b, p. 144).

The "near-miss" (nearly won) phenomenon may play a role in persistence characterised by over-commitment. Paradoxically, the failure of a near-miss may provide encouragement to persevere "by indicating that success may be within reach ... there was a noticeable tendency to think of gaining information from a near-miss even when the outcome could only be a matter of chance" (Reid, 1986, pp. 32–33). Griffiths (1990, 1991a) has suggested that frequent players will experience many near-misses, "the player is not constantly losing but constantly nearly winning" (Griffiths, 1999b, p. 442), possibly promoting the illusion of being due a win. It has also been suggested that near-misses might induce much regret if the alternative scenario of winning can easily be imagined (Kahneman & Tversky, 1982). Gambling immediately after a near-miss may be an attempt to eliminate the highly aversive feelings associated with regret (Loftus & Loftus, 1983; cited in Reid, 1986). Reid (1986) argued that it is possible to experience both excitement and encouragement, and frustration, in response to a near-miss. Heavily involved fruit-machine players have reported excitement at near-misses (Griffiths, 1991a). Browne (1989) observed that regular poker players are unlikely to play for 6 h without experiencing a distressing near-miss ("bad beat") in which a very good hand gets beaten against the odds, and that near-misses were a major reason for losing emotional control ("going on tilt") and consequently chasing losses.

Lesieur (1984) pointed out that, given the intermittent reinforcement of winning, and past experience of "winning streaks", it is not surprising that the "chasers" believe that a major recovery is possible providing there is sufficient capital to continue betting. He describes gambling as a unique behaviour in that it both creates a problem but also provides the means by which to resolve the problem.

There appear to be two major difficulties associated with cognitive theory as it pertains to chasing behaviour. The first is that cognitive errors are commonplace amongst gamblers (including those for whom gambling is non-problematic), so cognitive theory cannot claim to offer a complete explanation of excessive gambling (Ladouceur & Walker, 1996). Developments in cognitive theory that specify the conditions under which erroneous perceptions and faulty beliefs contribute to chasing behaviour and impaired control are required. Secondly, although there is some evidence that high-frequency gamblers are more likely to experience erroneous beliefs than are those who gamble infrequently, there is little evidence as yet to support the claims that cognitive biases and errors are indeed predictive of chasing and impaired control.

Although there have been several approaches to classifying gambling-related cognitions (Wagenaar, 1988; Griffiths, 1993a, 1994b; Toneatto et al.,

1997; Toneatto, 1999), only recently has a measure been developed. Raylu and Oei (2004) generated items to assess the three types of cognition commonly associated with gambling; beliefs in personal control, in an ability to predict gambling outcomes, and an interpretation bias (e.g. attributing wins to skill, losses to the influence of others or circumstances) and added two other categories drawn more broadly from the addiction literature, expectations of the effects of gambling and thoughts of inability to control gambling. The factor solution to their 23-item scale, the Gambling-Related Cognitions Scale (GRCS), supported this classification into five subscales that accounted for 70% of the variance. However, it was notable that the "impaired control" subscale (items such as "I can't function without gambling" and "I am not strong enough to stop gambling") predominated, accounting for 44% of the variance compared to the remaining four subscales, none of which reached 10%.

There is common ground between this work and that on passion and gambling by Rousseau et al. (2002) that specified two types of passion, obsessive and harmonious: the former subjectively experienced as an internal pressure to carry out a behaviour and the latter experienced as a controlled choice to engage in an activity known to give rise to pleasure and also to experience "fit", to be in harmony with other aspects and values in their life. Roussseau et al. (2002) reported on their work to validate a short version of the Passion Scale suitable for gambling. Commendably, they recruited casino gamblers ($N = 312$) in the venue (Montreal Casino) for a brief interview and included descriptive items concerning each respondent's gambling and demographics. The results of factor analyses confirmed that the two scales (five items in each) formed separate factors with the first, Obsessive Passion accounting for almost 40% of the variance, and the second, Harmonious Passion for less than 20%. The authors interpreted the weak Pearson correlation between the two scales of 0.28 ($N = 312$) as confirming their expectations of relative independence. Other psychometric characteristics were shown to be acceptable and the potential of the approach for future gambling research was claimed by the authors on the basis of unpublished work completed on the psychological basis of passion, for example its links to personality and to childhood development.

However, the most relevant results of the study to the present discussion are those that predicted level of involvement in gambling. Reporting partial correlations that controlled for the other scale, only the Obsessive Scale was strongly and significantly associated with the amount of money gambled and being a "heavy" gambler: "... *participants who reported higher levels of obsessive passion toward gambling also reported gambling with more money in general and perceived themselves as being heavier gamblers ...*" (p. 58).

If one then considers the items in the Obsessive Scale:

- I cannot live without this gambling game.
- I am emotionally dependent on this gambling game.
- I have a tough time controlling my need to play this gambling game.
- I have an almost obsessive feeling for this gambling game.
- The urge is so strong I cannot help myself from playing this gambling game.

The parallels with the work of Raylu and Oei (2004) are apparent. The problem facing the researcher is whether impaired control is considered as a cognitive–emotional variable, and if so does this then encompass all the related themes of beliefs in skill, control and maybe chasing too? As suggested in Chapter 2 when discussing the results for chasing (cognitive, emotional and behavioural components) and impaired control (O'Connor & Dickerson, 2003, 2003a), there is the possibility that all such cognitive themes may be secondary to the evolving emotional salience of gambling when the behaviour becomes a regular leisure activity (Boyer & Dickerson, 2003).

In recent research into the cognitive biases in the addictive behaviours generally, there has been a tendency to depend less on subjective self-report methods and rather to use objective assessment techniques such as the Stroop and word stem completion tasks (McCusker, 2001). Modified formats of the Stroop task (Stroop, 1935) have been used to study eating disorders (e.g. Green et al., 1999) and problem drinking (e.g. Stormark et al., 2000). Two studies have focused on gambling. McCusker and Gettings (1997) using recruits to gamblers' Anonymous found that these problem gamblers showed attentional bias towards gambling-related words compared with neutral and emotionally salient drug-related words. (Control groups of non-gamblers and the spouses of the problem gamblers did not show the effect.) Interestingly the effect was shown to very specifically linked to the current preferred form of continuous gambling: thus off-course betters showed a significantly stronger bias for words associated with that form of gambling (e.g. "horse", "racing", "jockey" rather than words such as "card", "twenty-one", "ace" that are associated with blackjack).

The second study by Boyer and Dickerson (2003) recruited current EGM players divided into high and low impaired self-control over gambling using the SGC (18-item version, Baron et al., 1995) found an attentional bias effect for words relating to gaming machine play (e.g. "jackpot", "credits", "payouts") compared with neutral and emotional drug-related words for the low control group only. Both studies interpreted their results within the automaticity paradigm account of the Stroop effect (Macleod, 1991; Tzelgov et al., 1997): the processing of addiction-related words is an automated process that depends on current emotional salience *and* training.

The Role of Coping

In their discussion article Dickerson & Baron (2000) comment that the relevance of coping to impaired control over gambling has been derived from the results for other addictive behaviours, in particular alcohol: the association between the use of avoidance coping strategies and poorer outcome of intervention (e.g. Moos et al., 1990) and the increased risk of harmful impacts (Simpson & Arroyo, 1998). More specific predictions about the role of coping in problem gambling were made from a social learning model (Sharpe & Tarrier, 1993; Sharpe, 2002). It was predicted that adaptive coping would enable regular gamblers to control urges to gamble, manage autonomic arousal and challenge irrational expectations of winning.

The published literature on coping and gambling provides modest support for the former broad associations with levels of risk and harm. McCormick (1994) found an association between emotion-focused coping and greater severity of gambling-related problems but incorrectly assumed this to indicate a style of coping, as a single situation specific measure of coping had been used. Di Dio and Ong (1997) surveyed EGM players and found that avoidance coping and current level of subjective stress accounted for 43% of the variance in the dependant variable of problem gambling. Unfortunately the coping scale they used was a collation of items from different measures and included some that were identical to some in the survey version of the DSM-IV (APA, 1994) criteria for pathological gambling that was the measure of the independent variable.

In a study of women EGM players (Scannell et al., 2000), low control over their gaming as measured by a short version of the SGC, Baron et al. (1995) reported higher levels of emotion-focused coping, especially avoidance in dealing with the specific situation, "the most stressful event of the last 3 years". Once again the authors incorrectly generalised from this that an avoidance style of coping had been shown to be associated with a style of gaming that showed poor self-control and rendered the player at great risk of harmful impacts arising from their gambling.

Critiquing these studies, Shepherd and Dickerson (2001) noted the lack of conceptual clarity in failing to specify the context in which the coping took place in terms of the type and controllability of the stressor (Folkman et al., 1986) or to use a measure with both situational and dispositional formats, for example the Coping Orientation to Problems Experienced (COPE; Carver et al., 1989).

Shepherd and Dickerson (2001) studied coping using the stressor *loss* and varied controllability in two ways: gambling losses using the within subject variable of high and low self-control of gambling (SGC, Baron et al., 1995), and secondly using two scenarios unconnected with gambling, one inherently controllable (inter-state employment move) the other uncontrollable (death of a friend from illness).

Using a short version of the COPE (Hudek-Knezevic & Kardum, 2005) to ensure survey completion in gaming venues, 226 EGM players (68% men) were recruited. The results strongly supported the expectation that EGM gamblers with low self-control over their gaming used significantly greater avoidance coping when facing gambling losses: for example "pretending the loss had not happened". Secondly, these low control players also were more likely to use avoidance coping in both controllable and uncontrollable loss situations unrelated to their gambling. Gender was not a significant influence on the selection of coping responses.

These results go some way to suggest that gamblers who are at high risk of the harmful impacts of gambling because of their low self-control over cash and time expenditure on gaming may have a stable, predominantly avoidance coping response to loss situations. Whether this confirms the possible developmentally acquired sensitivity to loss stressors (Whitman-Raymond, 1988) merits further study. Another question arising from the results of Shepherd & Dickerson (2001) was why the low self-control players also reported a high level of problem-solving coping, that is traditionally assumed to be adaptive, to the gambling losses. An example of one COPE item illustrates why the question could not be resolved: If "I made a plan of action to deal with the loss" was endorsed, it could mean either the player stopped playing and saved money to replace the loss (adaptive), or the player planned from whom to borrow money in order to continue gambling at the same level (a response likely to exacerbate the problem). The resolution of the question requires a coping item set designed specifically for gambling.

A Conceptual Basis for Modelling Impaired Self-Control of Gambling

The literature review was restricted in its scope to an examination of the psychological variables that had been shown to contribute to problem/pathological gambling and might therefore be expected to play a role in the erosion of self-control of gambling behaviour in non-clinical groups of regular gamblers who preferred continuous forms such as EGM play, off-course betting and casino table games.

The traditional assumption of the significant role of conditioning (e.g. Cornish, 1978) was endorsed but it was emphasised that the common operant assumptions were not supported. Adequate accounts of existing data may require cognitive conceptualisations of the learning process (e.g. the work of Vogel-Sprott & Fillmore, 1999) examining expectations within an associative learning model of drug taking). In discussing reinforcement in gambling strong positive emotional experience, its timing and relationship to the "fixed" sequence of stimuli comprising continuous forms of gambling was noted: the self-report and physiological recordings during actual gambling has demonstrated higher levels of such emotion for regular gamblers compared with infrequent or novice gamblers. Pre-existing state and trait factors such as dysphoric mood and individual differences, such as impulsivity or excitement-seeking, were also considered likely to contribute to impaired self-control over gambling.

Cognitive themes such as beliefs about skill, the illusion of control and the estimation of probabilities have all been shown to be strongly associated with regular and problem gambling, so much so that in some conceptual models (e.g. on passion and gambling by Rousseau et al., 2002) they have been integrated with beliefs and expectations about impaired self-control. Another aspect of regular and problem gambling, chasing, whether assessed in terms of beliefs, emotions or actual chasing behaviour, shows a very close association with independently assessed impaired control (O'Connor & Dickerson, 2003). Clearly a case can be made for including chasing, and perhaps other cognitive factors such as the illusion of control, in measures of impaired self-control. An alternative approach has been to include measures of impaired self-control as a subscale in a general measure of gambling cognitions (e.g. Raylu & Oei, 2004). Either course may run the risk of significantly reducing the importance of impaired control in the development of conceptual models of the addictive process in gambling as may have occurred in relation to the excessive consumption of alcohol. The results of the work around defining and measuring impaired self-control as a quantifiable dimension in its own right (as described in Chapter 2) was taken as support for a research focus on this factor as the key dependent variable. Whether cognitive factors such as the illusion of control, beliefs in skill, etc. are best considered components of impaired control, or variables that contribute to it, requires further examination.

4

Models of Impaired Self-Control of Gambling

Empirical Model of EGM Play

The beginning of Chapter 2 revisited the arguments summarised in the position article (Dickerson & Baron, 2000), the main theme of which was that future research into excessive gambling might examine the behaviour in terms of the construct of choice or subjective control, rather than as pathology or mental disorder. Not that this was to deny the harmful impacts or the mental disorder model but rather because this approach had the potential to be a more productive research frame of reference focusing on the key addictive construct of self-control. It also shifted the focus from clinical populations to people who were currently regular gamblers, engaged in a continuous form of gambling weekly or more often: a group that in the Australian context has been demonstrated to be most at risk of the harmful impacts of gambling. In the following research all participants were regular electronic gaming machines (EGM) players.

Chapter 3 reviewed the range of variables that may contribute to the development of impaired self-control and the figure below summarises those selected for empirical exploration in a sequence of two pilot studies exploring measures and methods and one main study. The first of the sequence was conducted in 1997, the second in 2001 and the final project data collection was completed at the beginning of 2002. The pilot studies were funded by research "seed" monies from the University of Western Sydney and the final project by the Casino Community Benefit Fund (a state government administered fund used to deliver services for problem gamblers and related research) following a peer evaluated competitive round of research funding. Much of the planning and data collection preceded some of the studies reviewed in the previous chapter and therefore does not incorporate all the insights nor address all the issues contained in that review.

The major variables predicting impaired control were prior or pre-existing negative emotion, coping styles, social support, personality and alcohol consumption.

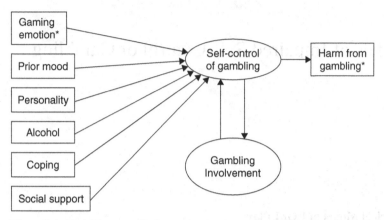

Figure 4.1. Variables contributing to the development of level of involvement and impaired control of gambling: exploratory stage. *Variable added at second pilot study.

The original illustration of the possible relationships (Dickerson & Baron, 2000) was very complex and the above simplification (Figure 4.1), aided by Baron & Kenny's (1986) clarification of moderator and mediator variables, shows the arrowed relationships as simple predictor variables of impaired control. The role of coping and social support could be conceptualised as directly preventing the erosion of self-control, but the evidence from the other addictive behaviours such as alcohol suggested that both contributed to maintaining the gains of treatment interventions, which in the context of a non-clinical group of regular gamblers might equate to moderating the development of harmful impacts.

The other predicted variable in the model was level of involvement in gaming machine play. It was also considered to have a circular relationship with impaired control, that is both act as predictor and predicted variables of each other. Level of involvement was suggested by Dickerson & Baron (2000) to contain three factors: expenditure, frequency or days per week of gambling (between sessions frequency) and duration of play (within session duration). However, this variable was not operationally defined and needed to be specified for empirical study. Level of involvement is a latent construct that was conceptualised as reflecting the way in which regular players differed from infrequent players (Cornish, 1978) and should indicate the extent of conditioning or learning. Behaviourally, for the majority of gamblers, this would be reflected in time spent playing gaming machines. Under this definition both days per week and duration of play constitute the best measure of level of involvement in gaming machine play. The gambler who plays more frequently and for longer periods of time can reasonably be considered more involved in their gambling than someone spending less time in front of the gaming machine. Expenditure fails as an adequate measure of level of involvement as it may merely reflect the gambler's disposable income rather than involvement in gaming machine play.

The two pilot studies (Haw & Dickerson, 2005) involved the "in venue" recruitment of two separate samples totalling 300 regular players. All were weekly or more frequent players and the two samples reported similar levels of impaired control. (The characteristics of each group are given at the footnote on p. 30) In the first study, significant correlations were found between impaired self-control and the predictor variables of prior negative mood, a general measure of neuroticism, coping and level of hazardous alcohol consumption. These variables did not correlate with level of involvement.

In the second study the predictions for personality were refined to be specific to impulsivity and excitement seeking. Also added was a measure of social support, rather than depending on the demographic data dichotomy of "partnered" versus "single". Also missing from the first model was any measure of the harmful impacts of gambling, the assumed outcome of impaired control. One additional predictor variable was added, emotion experienced during gaming. This had previously been implicated in impaired control of off-course betting (Dickerson et al., 1987) and there were emerging results supporting the application of recent human decision theory models to gambling such as regret theory (O'Connor, 2000) and subjective expected emotion (SEE) (Mellers et al., 1999).

The procedure differed from the first study only in that the incentive was paid with a pre-purchased store voucher immediately after completion of the questionnaire in the venue rather than by subsequent mail-out. This was done to better protect their anonymity and save time and research costs. Recruitment was more rapidly completed but data entry suggested strong response biases in some of the measures and lack of consistency in reported gambling involvement in particular. The group was somewhat younger than in the first and the proportion scoring in the "at risk" category on the South Oaks Gambling Screen (SOGS) was twice as high as expected (Productivity Commission, 1999).

Main Study (O'Connor et al., 2005)

The first study was a less than ideal platform to progress the modelling of impaired control (the results are discussed elsewhere; Haw & Dickerson, 2005). The principle conclusion drawn was the need to ensure that players

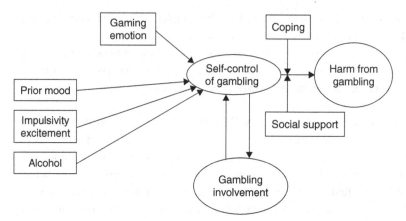

Figure 4.2. Variables contributing to the development of level of involvement and impaired control of gambling: main study.

recruited had sufficient involvement in the study to ensure consistent reporting. In the final study this was achieved by designing a prospective, continuing assessment of players over a 6-month period. This latter "follow-up" period was justified in the design as providing an opportunity to monitor changes in level of involvement and to qualitatively assess those players who reported the greatest changes, either increasing or decreasing their time spent gaming.

In the model for the main study (Figure 4.2) it was decided that the role of coping in moderating the development of impaired control could not be determined by a general measure of coping (see discussion at p. 80) but would need a scale specific to gambling (Shepherd & Dickerson, 2001). In the absence of such a measure it was predicted that coping would act as a moderator variable for the harm that could arise from impaired control over gambling. In the absence of more specific empirical data social support predictions were based on the generic descriptions of pathological gamblers where "the bail-out" by significant others plays a part in the development of the disorder (Custer, 1984) and therefore the variable was also expected to moderate the harmful impacts.

Prior negative mood, personality (specifically impulsivity and excitement seeking) and alcohol consumption were all predicted to contribute to the development of impaired self-control. Uncertainty remained whether for mood and personality the effect was a direct action or acted indirectly via an interaction with the emotion experienced during gaming. The role of negative mood in undermining self-control is well established in the addiction literature (Muraven & Baumeister,

2000) but a laboratory study suggested that for EGM play prior negative mood in regular players may enhance the level of positive emotion experienced during gaming (Hills et al., 2001). Impulsivity implies a "state" level of poorer self-control and would therefore be expected to predict impaired control directly (Vitaro et al., 1999); excitement seeking was possibly more complex acting via the intervening variable of gaming emotion (Leary & Dickerson, 1985; Dickerson et al., 1987).

Absent from the predictor variables were cognitive variables such as beliefs in winning, skill at gaming or chasing. As discussed earlier, although it is well established that such variables are implicated in problem gambling there were both conceptual and measurement reasons why they were not included at this stage of the investigation of impaired self-control. In particular, the detailed study of the emotional, cognitive and behavioural aspects of chasing O'Connor (2000) raised the question of whether these subjective reports of regular gamblers indicated the player's awareness of the evolving impairment of their self-control: that the construct of chasing was both a post hoc self-explanation of impaired self-control and a possible justification for continuing to gamble or returning to gamble again. Other cognitive themes such as expectations of winning and beliefs in skill could serve similar functions. Psychometric measures of cognitive aspects of gambling have been slow to emerge and the most recent, the Gambling-Related Cognition Scale (GRCS) (Raylu & Oei, 2004), includes items of self-control along with cognitive biases, expectations and illusions, albeit with some separation into subscales. Cognitive gambling variables were therefore not included amongst the independent variables at this stage.

Method

Participants

A convenience sample of 360 adult, regular poker machine players was initially recruited over three sessions and 4 days. Players were sampled from different times of the day and both weekdays and during the weekend. All participants were recruited from a single licensed club in Western Sydney, Australia, provided they played the poker machines "about twice a week" or more. Participants were informed that they would be required to complete a series of six telephone interviews over a period of approximately 6–7 months for which they would be paid a total of $50.00. Participants received their payment in the form of department store gift vouchers, $20.00 for participating in the first interview and $30.00 on completion of the fifth follow-up interview.

After initially being recruited, just over 40% either withdrew or did not respond to repeated calls. The final sample comprised 98 men and 114 women. The average participant was aged between 45- and 49-year old; however, the largest age group was the youngest age group, the 18–24 years ($n = 32$). The average household income of participants was between $40,000.00 and $50,000.00 though 50% of the sample had a household income of less than $40,000.00. The overwhelming majority (83%) of participants came from an English-speaking background and on average had a senior secondary level of education.

In terms of gambling patterns, the current sample gambled twice a week for about 2–2.5 h, spending on average $83.00 per session; however, 65% of the sample spent $50.00 or less per session and 3% spent $300.00 or more. The average participant had been gambling for 7 years with 50% of the sample gambling for more than 4 years.

Materials

As well as covering this descriptive information, a single survey instrument was developed to measure impulsivity, excitement seeking (the Excitement Seeking and Impulsivity sub-scales from the Revised NEO Personality Inventory (NEO-PI-R; Costa & McCrae, 1992a)), prior negative mood (Depression, Anxiety and Stress Scale (DASS); Lovibond & Lovibond, 1995), social support (Inventory of Socially Supportive Behaviours (ISSB); Barrera et al., 1981), coping strategies (short form of Frydenberg & Lewis', 1997 Coping Scale for Adults (CSA)), alcohol use (Alcohol Use Disorders Identification Test (AUDIT), World Health Organisation), self-control over gambling (Scale of Gambling Choices (SGC); Baron et al., 1995 but scored as the 12-item version), harmful impacts of gambling (Victorian Gambling Screen (VGS); Ben-Tovim et al., 2001) and affect during EGM play (4-point Likert scale (1, not at all to 4, very much so)) as to whether participants felt calm, tense, at ease and/or over-excited during "reel spin" (Leary & Dickerson, 1985). All variables were measured as they related to participant's experiences over *the last 6-months*.

Descriptive Results for Main Variables

The mean SGC score (there was no sex difference) was 24.0 (SD: 10.5, range: 12–58). At 6-month follow-up SGC scores correlated at 0.67. However, a paired sample t-test (i.e. sensitive to change on a case-by-case basis) revealed significantly different scores at follow-up ($t = 5.75$, d.f. $= 158$, $p < 0.000$). This is attributable to quite large shifts in impaired control across the sample, with 5.7% increasing their SGC scores by 6 or more, and 28.3% reducing their scores by 6 or more. A change of the magnitude of six points is considerable in that it was the difference between being categorised as having no problems and "possible problems" on the Harm Scale (i.e. a mean impaired control score of 17.5 compared to 23.8, respectively).

Largely consistent with earlier findings (O'Connor & Dickerson, 2003; Kyngdon, 2004), the SGC was found to be one factor, accounting for over half (53%) of all variance. However, the one factor was achieved after eliminating eight cases from analysis; these cases appeared to have impaired control scores that were an artefact of a response set (a failure to adjust to a change from items worded in the positive to four items worded in the negative produced extremely high scores across eight items and extremely low scores on four items, thus generating a second, uninterpretable, factor).

The mean VGS score (again there was no sex difference) was 14.2 (SD: 14.7, range 0–63). Almost one-quarter (24%) scored in the problem gambler category (21+), with another quarter (25%) scoring as possible problem gamblers (9–20). This compares with 15% of all regular gamblers who preferred continuous forms being classified as problem gamblers in the Productivity Commission's survey (1999). O'Connor et al. (2005) noted that the frequency of sessions was higher in their sample and that rates of expenditure were generally higher for EGM players. There was a very high correlation between impaired control scores and harm scores ($r = 0.80$).

The proportion (17.2%) scoring in the hazardous level for alcohol consumption and related problems (as measured by the AUDIT; scores >8) and the proportion that scored in *both* the problem gambler and the hazardous drinking category (12%) were similar but lower than the one other published data set for a similar group of regular EGM players (Dickerson et al., 2001).

Summary of Regression Analyses

The predictor variables provided a strong account of impaired self-control, accounting for over half the variance, with only excitement seeking failing to achieve significance (O'Connor et al., 2005). Separate regression analyses for men and women yielded interesting gender differences: for the male players impulsivity and levels of hazardous alcohol intake contrasted with the female players' prior negative mood (stress and depression). Common to both sexes was level of time involvement in gambling and strength of emotional engagement during EGM play. The combined predictor variables gave an adjusted r^2 of 0.46 and 0.58 for men and women, respectively.

Not surprisingly given the shifts in individual levels of impaired control, variables measured at baseline were not highly predictive of impaired control at follow-up and accounted for only 25% of the variance, but gaming emotion and level of involvement in gambling remained significant for both men and women, and prior negative mood remained significant for women.

Critical Comment on Methodology

Recruiting research participants in gambling venues is notoriously difficult. Nonetheless, during a period of about 5 years projects were completed in a number of venues, with different personnel and slightly different methods and incentives. In toto almost 1000 men and women regular players completed assessment measures and there have been fairly consistent findings for the key-dependent variable of impaired self-control (see p. 30). In this main study (O'Connor et al., 2005), despite the initial immediate attrition of 40% of those who volunteered a name and contact telephone number, of those who completed the first assessment 80% were retained through to the end of the project some 6 months later. As argued in the literature on the prevalence of problem gambling (e.g. Productivity Commission, 1999) it is likely that those regular players who have the most significant harmful impacts from gambling (those who are more likely to perceive themselves as problem gamblers) will avoid participation in such research, or if recruited will drop out. Thus problem gamblers/pathological gamblers are likely to be under represented in samples of regular players. Despite this, the sample in this main study recorded proportions of players experiencing significant harmful impacts somewhat greater than found elsewhere in the literature, although the differences may be attributable in part to the slightly different proportions generated by the VGS (Ben-Tovim et al., 2001) compared with the SOGS (Lesieur & Blume, 1987) (for a comparison see Gambling Research Panel (GRP), 2004).

Although the data was entirely self-reported, the measures have shown acceptable levels of reliability and validity, and the measure of the independent variable, impaired self-control (SGC-12 item), yielded a similar factor solution similar to the two previous independent studies (O'Connor & Dickerson, 2003; Kyngdon, 2004) once the eight subjects showing the most extreme response bias were excluded. The items measuring gaming emotion enabled participants to indicate the intensity of their feelings, but not the subjective valence (Hills et al., 2001). Future studies will need to address this weakness and also to distinguish session start from session end: as discussed earlier it is likely that the variables contributing to impaired self-control at each decision point will be subtly different.

Discussion of Empirical Findings

In this main study, despite these methodological concerns the results provide the first empirical steps in understanding the psychological processes that may lead to the impairment of self-control of gaming machine play, an impairment that is no ephemeral experience but is strongly associated with subsequent significant harmful consequences. In the non-clinical sample of regular players, current level of involvement in gaming and the intensity of the emotion during actual EGM play were significant predictors of the level of impaired self-control. For women players prior non-clinical levels of negative mood significantly increased the reported levels of impaired self-control. In contrast, in men it was the individual difference of impulsivity together with hazardous levels of alcohol consumption that were associated with higher impairment of self-control.

These gender differences match very similar findings for other addictive behaviours (Orford, 2001) and suggest rather different processes facilitate the erosion of self-control in men and women: for women gaming may be providing a period of mood repair or escape and for men the excitement/stimulation of an uncontrolled session of gambling behaviour. In clarifying these gender differences, measures of gaming emotion yielding both intensity and valence may show that for women "relaxation" and "calm" may contrast with "excitement" and "arousal" for men. In men the results match the prospective findings for adolescent gamblers (Vitaro et al., 1999) and in the same paper the authors identify four aspects of the individual difference that might comprise the mechanism by which impulsivity contributes to impaired control: (1) excessive responsiveness to positive outcomes, (2) quick responding with little consideration of consequences, (3) insensitivity to negative/punishing outcomes and (4) poorer inherent levels of general self-control.

The level of impairment of self-control for the group as a whole remained relatively stable over a period of 6 months yielding a test–retest correlation of 0.68 for the SGC, but this taken alone would fail to take into account the proportion of players whose level of self-control changed significantly over this period, 8% increasing their impairment by a considerable amount and almost 20% decreasing. This process of relatively rapid change matches similar results for regular video lottery players in Nova Scotia (Schellinck & Schrans, 1998) and may underpin the similar observations in follow-up studies of survey-identified pathological gamblers (Abbott et al., 1999). Certainly the picture of the self-control of some regular players is one of dynamic tension, perhaps a continual adjusting and readjusting in response to the facilitating variables of negative moods, perhaps heightened gaming emotion following a large win, the accrual of debts following a particularly uncontrolled session of play, and so on.

Theoretical Speculations

The results of the main study were entirely predictable from the existing literature on problem gambling reviewed in Chapter 3, but it is the context of the findings that is unique. The dependent variable was not problem or pathological gambling but the psychological construct of impaired self-control of gambling. Impairment of self-control has consistently been shown to be a common experience of regular gaming machine players (and probably of other continuous forms of gambling) and the results of O'Connor et al. (2005) demonstrated that normal, non-pathological, psychological variables provide a strong account of how this impairment may be generated.

That the predictor variables common to both men and women were level of involvement and the intensity of emotion experienced during gambling, and these variables remained significant predictors of impaired control 6 months later, is suggestive of a learning process, a process commonly assumed (e.g. Cornish, 1978) but typically rejected on the erroneous assumption that only a small proportion of regular gamblers show the assumed detrimental effects of conditioning (e.g. Blaszczynski & Nower, 2002; Aasved, 2003; Blaszczynski et al., 2004). The importance of frequency of sessions and session length must not be underestimated, as significant results for this variable were shown despite restricting the range to twice weekly sessions of gambling or more.

If the putative conditioning process is conceptualised in terms of expectations, then it is relevant to pose the question: to what extent would the subjective expectations of emotion (i.e. emotion during gambling) contribute to an account of impaired self-control? Such a model (SEE) has been demonstrated to provide a strong account of gambling choices in the laboratory (Mellers et al., 1999). In the present context it would be predicted that such a cognitive variable might absorb much of the variance currently attributed to other more specifically "problem gambling" cognitive variables such as expectations of winning, illusions of skill/control and possibly even the cognitive–emotional aspects of chasing.

Such speculations derive from the implicit assumption that the primary source of what has been identified as the core defining characteristic of problem and pathological gambling, impaired self-control (e.g. Blaszczynski & Nower, 2002), is the essentially normal process of conditioning; several hours each week of repetitive sequences of gaming stimuli and rewarding intense emotion. If this is the origin of the addictive process in gambling, then it is entirely in keeping with the rest of the literature on addiction that such a process is enhanced in women by pre-existing non-clinical levels of negative mood and in men by trait impulsivity and hazardous levels of alcohol consumption. Whether impairment of self-control is a function of the availability of a specific control strength or resource (Muraven and Baumeister, 2000), or more directly determined by the strength of the conditioning itself, remains an important research question. Intuitively, if the level of impaired self-control is a function of the strength of conditioning then it seems unlikely that a specific "muscle" (Muraven and Baumeister, 2000) would evolve to counteract such a fundamental process.

Modelling Impaired Self-Control: A Model of Gambling Temptation–Restraint

In Chapter 2 the qualitative work of Maddern (2004) reported on the different ways in which young men and women who gambled regularly set limits to facilitate self-control. This she described in terms of a Limit Maintenance Model (LMM) and specified three different processes:

1. A unique group of self-regulated gamblers who did not consciously set limits but recognised it when it was reached. This absence of a need to set limits was interpreted in terms of dynamic self-regulation (Pintrich, 2000) in which intrinsically motivated values consistent with other broad themes of activity readily over-ride the urge to continue to gamble.
2. A self-regulated group who specified a limit knowing that they were at risk of gambling more than they preferred, occasionally revised it once only, and then abided by it.
3. A group who were described as contingency regulated, as it required some event such as expenditure of all cash in hand or venue closure for a session to end.

The psychological processes involved in the latter group was explained with reference to the Limit Violation Effect (Collins et al., 1994) as the qualitative analysis revealed two themes: a cognitive preoccupation with maintaining control and dysphoric mood arising from previous failures to maintain self-control over gambling.

Thus in developing the LMM, Maddern became increasingly aware that several of the cognitive, limit-setting themes and their linkages with emotional responses were very similar to constructs in the literature that have lead to the development of the conceptual model of temptation and restraint by Collins and her colleagues (Temptation and Restraint Inventory (TRI); Collins et al., 1994, 1997; Connors et al., 1998). Sharing the view that there are common psychological pathways involved in addictive behaviours (e.g. Orford, 2001) and of the need for gambling research to build conceptual bridges with existing psychological models (Dickerson & Baron, 2000), Maddern (2004) set out to examine the validity of the temptation and restraint model for gambling.

The question addressed was whether the factor structure, particularly the superordinate theme of temptation and restraint, of the alcohol TRI could be replicated for youth gamblers and whether the equivalent predictive associations would be found for levels of involvement in gambling and for the harmful impacts of gambling.

Measure: The Gambling Temptation and Restraint Inventory

Based on the alcohol TRI and following pilot work with groups of youth gamblers the Inventory comprised (followed by item number):

Govern:

Do you find that once you start gambling it is difficult for you to stop? (9)

Do you have difficulty controlling your gambling? (13)

Do you find that it takes considerable effort to keep your gambling under control? (15)

Emotion:

When you feel unhappy or anxious are you more likely to gamble? (1)

When you feel lonely are you more likely to gamble? (2)

Do you ever feel so stressed or nervous that you really need to gamble? (6)

Cognitive preoccupation:

Do you attempt to cut down the amount of time or money that you gamble? (4)

Do thoughts about gambling intrude into your everyday activities? (7)

Is it hard to distract yourself from thinking about gambling? (11)

Restrict:

How often do you attempt to cut down the amount you gamble? (3)

Do feelings of guilt about gambling too much help you control your gambling? (10)

Do you ever cut back on your gambling in an attempt to change your gambling habits? (14)

Concern:

Does seeing other people gamble remind you of your efforts to control your own gambling? (5)

Does seeing commercials, magazine advertisements, and or signs for gambling venues make you think about your need to limit your gambling? (8)

Do the sights and sounds of gambling make you think of limiting your gambling? (12)

(Respondents used a 1–9 scale from "never" to "always".)

Data Collection

In November 1999, Woolcott Research were contracted to conduct a random telephone survey of 800 men and women aged between 16 and 24 years in Sydney and New South Wales (NSW) country areas: the sample approximated population strata for age, sex and area (27,000 calls were made with a refusal rate of 10%).

The complete survey included demographic items, current gambling involvement of time and money, the Gambling Temptation and Restraint Inventory (G-TRI), the Harm scale (Productivity Commission, 1999), but the latter was given only to regular gamblers (gambling on continuous forms twice or more per month). (Based on the experience of the qualitative study, the Harm items were reframed asking respondents to the extent to which their gambling and a particular harm "was associated/went together" and if so how strongly. Pilot testing revealed that respondents interpreted the questions as asking the extent to which gambling caused the harms, whereas the original format tended to be rejected with respondents giving few item endorsements at all.)

High-school students were excluded from the telephone survey and the same instrument in a written format was administered to a random selection of six high schools in March 2000.

Sample Characteristics

Combining the two samples gave a total group of 1008 young people (51.5% female), mean age 19 years (SD = 2.52), 60% single/without current partner, 74.5% living at home with parent(s) and 20% were from non-English-speaking backgrounds.

Respondents who gambled 2–3 times per month were combined with those who gambled weekly and more often to form a group of 226 "regular" gamblers, representing 22.4% of the original sample, and the analysis of the G-TRI was based on the responses of this group.

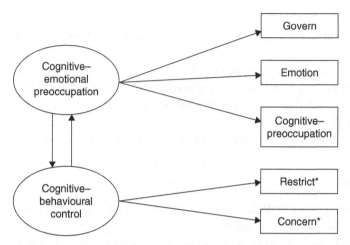

Figure 4.3. Schema of the Temptation–Restraint model (Collins & Lapp, 1992).
*These two factors/scales collapsed together plus item 4 from cognitive preoccupation in the Gambling TRI analysis.

Regular gambler group: two-thirds were aged 18 years and older, 64% were male and were more likely to be Sydney-based than country, NSW. Median spend per session of gambling was about $20.00 with slightly lower levels for under 18 years of age but half that level for female gamblers (the average spend per session for all players was $42.00).

The ratings of the 26 Harm items were normally distributed with only one item, "living situation issues" nominated by more than 10% of the group of regular gamblers (12.8%). Over 18 years were more significantly more likely than the younger gamblers (illegal in NSW) to have confirmed an association between their gambling and thoughts of suicide, fights with friends, taking money without asking and failure to repay borrowed money. There were also significant gender differences with males confirming the association between their gambling and losing/changing schools or jobs, lying to people, fighting with friends, relationship difficulties, shortage of money, borrowing money and problems with living situation.

The most recent modelling of the TRI completed by Collins and colleagues for alcohol specifies five scales supporting the key second-order constructs of cognitive–emotional preoccupation (CEP) and cognitive–behavioural control (CBC), and this model (Figure 4.3) was taken as the a priori schema for statistical testing.

The following stages of statistical analyses were completed for the G-TRI:

1. Five individual scales. (The one-factor congeneric solutions for each of the G-TRI scales yielded acceptable fit indices but final acceptability of the five-factor structure was decided by Confirmatory Factor Analysis (CFA).)
2. Scales were multi-dimensional but CFA resulted in a preferred four-factor solution, collapsing concern and restrict plus the addition of item 4 from cognitive preoccupation see Maddern (2004) (Table 30, p. 230).
3. Two second-order factors with the anticipated relationship were confirmed using structural equation modelling (second-order SEM).
4. Each of the second-order factors was validated using regression modelling: CBC predicted lower levels of gambling participation and harmful impacts, and CEP predicted higher levels of both.

The results provided broad support for the alcohol-derived model: four separate scales were supported by the data from the regular youth gamblers, with the concern and restrict scales collapsed together with the addition of item 4 from the cognitive preoccupation scales. The key second-order constructs were confirmed and validated.

Thus Maddern concluded that "the G-TRI results support the theoretical stance that the psychological processes underlying regular gambling embody dynamic tensions between temptation resulting in excessive levels of gambling and attempts at restriction. CEP with gambling was a risk factor for higher levels of gambling and CBC was associated with lower involvement in gambling and fewer reported impacts".

Gamblers at greater risk of the negative consequences arising from their gambling more typically gambled to escape negative emotions and were preoccupied with thoughts of gambling or limiting their gambling. In Maddern's opinion, the G-TRI captured the characteristics of that group that she had studied in detail qualitatively (see summary in p. 34). In particular, the driving force of the abstinence violation effect (AVE) was typified by those gamblers who set and then revised their session limits several times; some of the youth gamblers studies stated that it was less stressful to lose all their available money early in the session and "get it over with" rather than struggle with limits knowing that eventually they would fail. The G-TRI also made sense of the apparently anomalous position of the small group of gamblers in the qualitative study that named no limits and yet who seemed most controlled. In the context of restraint theory they had no preoccupation with gambling or setting limits and were not subject to the AVE.

Maddern noted the methodological limitations of her study, in particular the need for future explorations of the model to use a larger pool of items from which more stable factors can be developed. Nonetheless, the successful application of restraint theory to regular youth gamblers demonstrated the validity of generalising an established theoretical account of an addictive aspect of alcohol consumption to another addictive behaviour, gambling. Similar cognitive–behavioural processes seem to account for the problem of self-control encountered in the regular consumption of alcohol and continuous forms of gambling. Maddern's results for regular youth gamblers is entirely compatible with the notion of limited cognitive resources that enable self-control or the attainment of goals (Baumeister, 1997; Muraven & Baumeister, 2000; Pintrich, 2000), that is being cognitively preoccupied with gambling, setting limits, worries of breaking set limits, predispose the regular gambler to lose control.

Discussion of the Two Approaches to Exploring Impaired Self-Control

There is much in common to the two studies that set out to examine the ways in which gamblers attempt to maintain preferred levels of involvement of time and money expenditure. Both emphasised the importance of studying people who currently gamble regularly on continuous forms, O'Connor et al. (2005) selecting EGM players who gambled twice per week or more frequently and Maddern (2004), with the inclusion of 16–18-year-old students who have lower consumption patterns, settling for a minimum frequency of fortnightly, but with almost half gambling weekly or more.

In the overall context of the arguments in this monograph, it must be emphasised that such populations of gamblers only emerge as a significant proportion of the general population (e.g. 11% weekly EGM players in NSW Australia; Dickerson et al., 1998) where there is convenience access to continuous forms of gambling. Where such populations do emerge, they account for over 85% of the total expenditure on their preferred form of gambling (Dickerson et al., 1998) and are the gambling consumer group most at risk of significant harmful impacts arising from their gambling (approximately one in five; Productivity Commission, 1999). Therefore the results from the study of such regular gamblers will have significant implications for all aspects of gambling policy in jurisdictions which now or in the future have, or intend to have, convenience access to continuous forms of gambling such as EGMs, off-course betting and casino table games. An exploration of these implications is developed in the subsequent chapters.

Maddern's (2004) quantitative study demonstrated the value of research planned within a specific theoretical framework. The successful generalisation of a measure derived from restraint theory provides support for a wholly psychological conceptualisation of the addictive behaviours (e.g. Orford, 2001). In contrast, O'Connor et al. (2005) was essentially an empirical examination of the psychological variables that contribute to impaired self-control of gambling. The study did not address a specific theoretical question but selected key variables on the basis of existing evidence and theory, and as an initial broad exploratory study did provide evidence that may clarify which psychological processes may contribute to the erosion of self-control common to the addictive behaviours.

Taken together both studies show some progress has been made towards the realisation of the theoretical and research goals anticipated in the position paper of Dickerson & Baron (2000): by means of a focus on a more homogeneous psychological-dependent variable than pathological gambling, albeit the complex one of impaired self-control, to progress research towards better integration of gambling research with the addictions and also with the discipline of psychology itself.

5

Implications for Treatment Approaches to Problem Gambling Arising from the Model of Impaired Control

"Responsible gambling" has become the internationally accepted way of referring to all policies and strategies that have as their goal the prevention and amelioration of the harmful impacts arising from gambling (Productivity Commission, 1999). This includes:

1. Direct treatment of client problem gamblers and their families.
2. Harm minimisation initiatives.
3. Community awareness campaigns.

The following sequence of chapters briefly examines the possible implications of the measurement and modelling of impaired control for the treatment of problem gamblers (this chapter), for harm minimisation (Chapter 6) and in the case study of Victoria (Chapter 7) provides a working illustration of the integration of the broad range of strategies.

Do Existing Treatments Work? Conclusions from Treatment Literature Reviews

Recent reviews of the literature describing the treatment of problem and pathological gamblers have tended to be somewhat optimistic about the efficacy of the available methods (Lopez Viets & Miller, 1997; Victorian Department of Human Services (DHS), 2000; GRP, 2003a). This must be tempered by the findings of Oakley-Browne & Mobberly (2002) who, in applying the rigorous criteria of the Cochrane Review, found only four randomised controlled trials. They were only able to conclude that there was a lack of evidence for the effective treatment of pathological gambling but that cognitive–behavioural interventions were more effective than control treatments for both short- and long-term outcome evaluations (e.g. Ladouceur et al., 2001).

The two independent reviews completed in Australia cast a wider net and included individual case studies and service delivery descriptions in their process of evaluation. The first of these (O'Connor et al., 2000) was completed by a team from one of the three addiction centres of excellence, The National Centre for Education and Training on Addiction (NCETA) at Flinders University, a centre with considerable experience in evaluating the internationally published treatment outcome research of addictive behaviours (e.g. Kamieniecki et al., 1998).

The methodology for the literature search was specified and included a standardised word trail to ensure consistency and that the reliability of the rating of selected papers was satisfactory. The literature review was considered in the broad theoretical context of the bio-psychosocial model (Green & Shellingberger, 1991), and given the needs of the DHS, efficacious interventions were then examined in the context of criteria relevant to human service delivery: affordability, availability, accessibility, sustainability and whether ethical and equity standards were satisfied.

The authors noted the general limitations in methodology, such as few randomised trials and the failure to use "blind" evaluations or collateral reports at follow-up, but nevertheless concluded that: *"there is currently a clear rationale, based on consistently reasonable outcomes with gambling and other excessive behaviours, coupled with robust theory, for utilising an array of cognitive–behavioural interventions such as cognitive restructuring, desensitisation procedures, problem solving and skills rehearsal, self-monitoring and relapse prevention."* (O'Connor et al., 2000: p. vii)

The report went on to suggest that such methods could be delivered in a *"reasonably cost-effective and affordable manner by a wide array of health professionals, after relevant training, in a variety of settings. Outpatient treatment appears to deliver comparable results to more intensive, inpatient residential treatment...."* (p. vii)

The most recent review (GRP, 2003a) critically appraised 64 reports of interventions with pathological gamblers and reached very similar conclusions: *"there appears support for ... using cognitive–behaviourally oriented approaches and multimodal approaches, delivered in community-based generalist agencies."* (p. 7)

The Bio-psychosocial Model as a Basis for Treatment

The bio-psychosocial model most closely linked to a cognitive–behavioural model of gambling and related interventions is that of Sharpe (2002). This

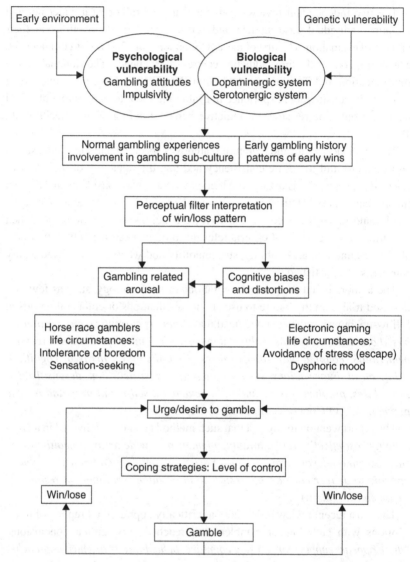

Figure 5.1. Bio-psychosocial model of pathological gambling (Sharpe, 2002).

model is reproduced in Figure 5.1 and clearly has much in common with the pathways model of Blaszczynski and Nower (2002). Contrary to a recent review (Aasved, 2003), there does seem to be a fairly general acceptance of the multicausal nature of problem gambling.

Sharpe (2002) uses the model not only to bring together a wide range of causal themes but also to outline the main treatment themes for interventions with problem gamblers. These are identified in the context of the need to clinically adapt the emphasis to the needs of each client.

The primary aims are to stop the gambling and to break the associations between the gambling behaviour and the cues associated with gambling, within and "outside" the venue, for example media reports, advertising, form guides. The methods to achieve this are initial restrictions on access to funds and venues and desensitisation (McConaghy et al., 1983) involving the imaginal rehearsal of venue visits and losing outcomes. In addition, the more typical range of cognitive–behavioural themes are identified: challenging irrational beliefs, supported by information about probabilities of winning and losing, reducing impulsive behaviours and problem-solving methods of coping.

In the longer term additional broad themes are noted, such as a "functional analysis" to assist the client to understand the role played by gambling in their life and the identification of relapse predictors, especially depressed mood.

Implications of the Model of Impaired Control for Treatment Methods

In the previous chapter impaired control of gaming machine play in regular players was shown to be driven by higher levels of involvement, stronger emotion during the process of gaming for both men and women, and prior non-clinical levels of negative mood in women and impulsivity and alcohol excess in men. In the absence of specific measures of cognitions, it was speculated that expectations of emotions rather than gambling outcomes might confirm the primary role of emotions, suggesting a less significant role for irrational beliefs about gambling in the erosion of self-control.

The first question is whether this account may be generalised to the problem gambler attending treatment. Although one in four regular electronic gaming machine (EGM) players scored in the "at risk" category, this group, by definition, is not a clinical group. It seems likely from the validation study of the Victorian Gambling Screen that one difference may be that such "at risk" regular players currently report *greater* pleasure from their gambling than either infrequent players or actual problem gamblers (Ben-Tovim et al., 2001). Thus, if problem gamblers report lower levels of pleasure, does this mean that the impaired control they experience has different origins? In terms of the within session dynamics, this seems unlikely because a loss of the positive emotional experience during play would suggest that the behaviour would not be maintained. However, amongst problem gamblers seeking treatment, one difference would likely be greater and more frequent negative moods such as guilt, frustration and depression occurring "between" sessions, perhaps arising from the greater level of harmful impacts amongst those seeking treatment. Thus, the model based on regular players may underestimate the impact of prior negative mood on impaired control. These possible differences temper the implications for improving interventions.

In the model (Figure 1 from Sharpe, 2002) above, it appears that self-control over gambling involvement is linked to coping strategies with problem solving approaches improving and sustaining control. If one of the main contributors to impaired control is the strength of positive emotion experienced during the process of gaming, then as long as the player is enjoying their gaming it is difficult to see how any coping strategy can be effective while play is ongoing (i.e. assuming EGMs function as they do currently). The coping to be effective would need to undermine or limit the levels of enjoyable emotion and this is counterintuitive in the consumption of an entertainment product such as gambling.

Nonetheless, the modelling of impaired control strongly supports the treatment goal prioritised by Sharpe (2002), the breaking of the learnt association between gambling cues and the emotional responses experienced while gambling. If, as may be the case for other addictive behaviours, the conditioning of the strong emotional salience of the gambling cues is a significant factor in gambling occurring without conscious control/monitoring (Coventry & Hudson, 2001; Boyer & Dickerson, 2003), in vivo cue exposure may be the most effective intervention technique (Tolchard & Battersby, 1996). The preferred method identified by Sharpe (2002) is desensitisation (McConaghy et al., 1983) that includes an exposure element in addition to learning alternative coping strategies such as relaxation and cognitive rehearsal of resisting gambling.

The cognitive–behavioural model also focuses on the significance of prior negative mood, one of the most common contributors to impaired control of addictive behaviours (Muraven & Baumeister, 2000) and confirmed for women gamblers in the modelling of EGM players. If regular players do use sessions to cope with stress (Sharpe, 2002) or to repair mood (Hills et al., 2001), this may inform preventative coping strategies for problem gamblers in treatment: they may be helped to identify and develop alternative activities that address this emotional need.

If future research confirms the role of anticipated emotions in impaired control this would emphasise emotions as the core theme in the addictive process rather than cognitions about probabilities of winning, skill and other illusory or irrational beliefs. The latter may then be seen as primarily providing the player with post hoc explanations of their own behaviour and personally and socially more acceptable ways of expressing their reasons for returning to gamble again. Qualitative research (that did not specifically focus on cognitions about winning) confirms that women in particular readily identify the emotional needs addressed by their gambling (DHS, 2000; O'Connor et al., 2000). Should research confirm these speculations, then interventions may need to include cognitive–emotional skills for problem gamblers: the identifying of emotions, emotional needs and adaptive ways of satisfying them while at the same time learning to have a less dependent relationship on gambling. It is likely that many skilled clinicians already seek to do this as part of their eclectic repertoire of interventions, but this has yet to be documented and evaluated.

Implications for Treatment Goals

In the modelling of impaired control the third variable implicated was level of involvement in gambling itself. Amongst regular players of EGMs, some level of reported impairment of self-control was very common and the erosion of control was envisaged as an ongoing process, an integral component of such continuous forms of gambling. This raises questions about whether treated problem gamblers should be advised that controlled gambling is a possible successful outcome of intervention.

Controlled gambling has generally been accepted as a satisfactory outcome of treatment (Lopez Viets & Miller, 1997; O'Connor et al., 2000; GRP, 2003a) and from the mental disorder model accepted at least for the "excessive" or "early stage" problem gambler if not for those who are highly dependent (Aasved, 2003). One case study using controlled gambling as a "method" of intervention (Dickerson & Weekes, 1979), illustrates some of the issues. The client problem gambler, wishing to continue to bet on horse racing learnt to place a limited set of selected bets prior to the start of racing on a non-working day and to leave the off-course venue without listening to the race broadcasts. He thereby changed a continuous form of gambling into a discontinuous one, retaining his regular interest and enjoyment of horse racing betting. This may be similar to the ways in which a person with eating disorders may learn to eat in a controlled fashion in specific situations or the person whose use of alcohol is hazardous may select a "safe" environment in which to drink after a period of abstinence. However, as all gambling on continuous forms takes place in regulated gambling venues (i.e. except Internet gambling) it is often not possible to alter the manner of gambling, to adopt a more controlled approach. The problem gambler attempting to play EGMs in a more controlled manner post-treatment would be involved in the same process that has been suggested erodes his or her self-control.

It may be that this process occurs in stages with the strongest impact being within the session of gaming itself, leading the player to play for longer. Subsequently, the impact of slowly deteriorating self-control might extend, precipitating additional sessions. In the follow-up of a minimal intervention, this pattern of changes was recorded during follow-up (Dickerson et al., 1990). These possibilities should not lead to a rejection of controlled gambling as a satisfactory treatment outcome, but rather to emphasise the need to independently assess exactly what is meant by "controlled". This should include the current level of involvement by product(s) consumed and confirmed by a collateral. Where regular gambling on a continuous form was reported this would need especially careful appraisal before "controlled" could be confirmed. The changes in the drinking status, from one period of follow-up to another in the evaluation of a very small number of treated alcoholics, can be taken as a salutary lesson (Davies, 1962; Edwards, 1985).

The common co-occurrence of gambling and alcohol problems, particularly in male gamblers, is a therapeutic complication well anticipated by most authors advising on treatment design (e.g. Blaszczynski, 1998; Pavalko, 2001; Sharpe, 2002). Its impact on the various tasks of the gambler seeking to re-establish self-control may be diverse and cannot be limited to excessive consumption; the evidence suggests that even, "safe" levels of alcohol consumption (Pols & Hawks, 1991) are associated with an inability to refrain from gambling (Baron & Dickerson, 1999) and greater persistence when losing (Kyngdon & Dickerson, 1999). In many jurisdictions gambling and alcohol are available in the same venue and the "mix" is commonly portrayed as the ideal, entertaining night out. There is no doubt that the goal of post-treatment controlled gambling may be particularly difficult to sustain for the individual who drinks alcohol, even at socially acceptable, "safe" levels. In terms of outcome evaluation this aspect requires careful assessment.

6

Implications for Harm Minimisation in the Management of Problem Gambling: Making Sense of "Responsible Gambling"

Harm Minimisation and Gambling

Harm minimisation has typically been defined as having the goal of reducing the *"adverse health, social and economic consequences of drug (gambling) use without necessarily requiring abstinence . . . Harm reduction is pragmatic and humanistic, focused on harms and priority issues."* (Centre for Addiction and Mental Health in Canada, cited by Blaszczynski et al., 2001). Harm reduction includes a wide variety of strategies, ranging from public health oriented preventatives through to clinical interventions that focus on low-risk behaviours.

The application of the concept to gambling has possibly broadened the range of preventative strategies, which for gambling include consumer complaints mechanisms, codes for responsible marketing, gambling venue staff training, gambling information pamphlets, restricting venue placement of ATMs, design of gaming machine features and venue self-exclusion procedures. Noting that the terms of reference in which any social debate is framed may determine the scope and freedom in which policy debate can develop, Korn et al. (2003) argued that there were benefits from viewing gambling as a public health matter: *"The value of a public health perspective is that it applies different 'lenses' for understanding gambling behaviour, analyzing its benefits and costs as well as identifying multilevel strategies and points of intervention."* (p. 236)

In this regard, the two national studies released in 1999, one from the USA and the other from Australia, provide a striking illustration of how limiting the debate to a preferred frame of reference or "lens" constricts the policy debate. In the USA the National Research Council (NRC, 1999) literature review was intended to *exclude* any harmful impacts that were not directly concerned with the mental disorder of pathological gambling. Consequently, the resulting reports (i.e. of

The National Gambling Impact Study Commission, the Final Report and the literature review, "Pathological Gambling: a Critical Review", by the NRC, 1999) had very little to say about harm minimisation strategies, reflecting a constricted gambling debate and perhaps mirroring the continuing rejection of such approaches in the areas of drug and alcohol addiction in the USA (Aasved, 2003). In contrast, the Productivity Commission (1999) reviewed the benefits and costs of the range of different approaches to defining and describing gambling and its psychological, social and economic impacts. Whole sections were devoted to consumer protection, which detailed harm minimisation strategies and recommended an evidence-based research evaluation of those strategies most likely to be effective in reducing problem gambling and least likely to disrupt the pleasure of non-problem gamblers.

Nonetheless, it seems that ideas have ways of subverting barriers and harm minimisation has entered the debate in the USA and internationally, but under the rubric of "responsible gambling". Used originally by the American Gaming Association "responsible gaming" programmes were *"Any strategy, policy or program instituted by a gaming company to proactively address problem gambling and/or underage gambling issues."* (AGA, 1998, pp. 1–7) Problem gambling was defined in terms of harm (e.g. Dickerson et al., 1998) and strategies dealt with:

1. venue staff training in awareness of problem gambling and how to act should players self-identify as having problems;
2. consumer programmes educating about gambling products, the possible harmful impacts and ways of obtaining help;
3. preventing underage gambling.

Since that time, "responsible gambling" has been used almost synonymously with harm minimisation, perhaps preferred by both governments and the industry in Australasia and Canada. It also covers the possible proactive strategies of all parties, governments, industry and the consumer/gambler. There are possible objections to the term being applied to gamblers (it could easily suggest that problem gamblers have nobody but themselves to blame for acting "irresponsibly"), but given that "responsible gambling" is the currently established term, it is used here despite a preference for the descriptor "low-risk gambling".

Rarely have definitions of "responsible gambling" been specified in ways that facilitate evidence-based evaluation, but the current definitions of responsible gaming by the Victorian Gaming Machine Industry (VGMI), a group that set international benchmarks with its Code of Practice, was an exception and illustrates the different applications to industry and the gambler:

"The industry's role (*i.e. the responsible provision of gaming*) is to offer products and services in a way that facilitates customers' ability to engage in responsible gaming."

and

"Responsible gaming is each person exercising a rational and sensible choice based on his or her individual circumstance."

The discussion will return to these definitions as a way of testing and clarifying the implications of the research on impaired control for the application of "responsible gambling" strategies.

The Productivity Commission (1999) carefully reviewed "responsible gambling" strategies worldwide and tabled 24 as "options for harm minimisation and prevention" (P. 16.88, Table 16.15). The strategies can be roughly classified into three main themes:

1. To educate the community and in particular the player so that there is a sound knowledge of the different types of gambling products and an awareness of the possible harmful impacts.
2. To ensure that problem/pathological gamblers were protected from further harmful gambling.
3. To render the process of gambling safer for all consumers.

Educational Strategies

Information about gambling and its impacts has included community awareness campaigns, signs and pamphlets targeting gamblers while they are in venues and training courses for venue staff to enable them to fulfil their role in the "responsible" provision of gambling. The primary goal of the community campaigns have been to sensitise the public to the fact that problems can and do arise from the gambling behaviour of some individuals, that these problems may be very severe and distressing for both the gambler and those involved in their life, and that services are available to assist with such problems. In Australasia, the latter have typically focused on a toll-free, confidential telephone help line, linked with access to locally available counselling services. (Examples of these themes are included in the chapter describing the "case example" of Victoria, Chapter 7, p. 124.)

The Productivity Commission report (1999) includes interesting examples of the types of information that may be helpful to gamblers, as well as reporting some very interesting interactions with industry groups who objected to illustrative examples given in the draft report. For example, in discussing the ways in which the consumer might best be advised of the probability of winning the big prize option on the electronic gaming machine (EGM) called the "Black Rhino": "*if they bet one line per button push, in order to have just a fifty per cent chance of getting 5 rhinos . . . it would take them 6.7 million button presses; or at ordinary rates of playing, it will take them 188 years of playing . . .*" (P. 16.17) The industry objected on the grounds that these examples showed a lack of understanding about how random number generators work, or the independence of outcomes, but these challenges were easily rebutted by the Commission, an independent group of well credentialed researchers, statisticians and economists.

Another very important example of the type of player information that could be made available was based on another current popular machine, the "Fast Fortune". This is available within New South Wales (NSW) at five different return rates ranging from 87.7 to 94.99 (i.e. for the hypothetical sample of 5 million plays for every dollar staked the machine will return 87.7 cents, etc.). The Commission noted that the true price of each is one minus the return rate and therefore the lowest return rate is 146% more expensive than the highest. "*Put another way, a person playing a 20 cents 'Fast Fortune' machine with 3 lines and one credit per button push, can expect to lose $21.64 on the 94.99 per cent machine and $53.14 a hour on the 87.7 per cent machine, though in all other respects the machines appear to be the same.*" (P. 16.13)

There have been attempts to develop a "Players' Charter" to indicate what information should be made available to anyone who consumes gambling products, but there has been no programme of research to evaluate how such information would be understood by the general public or whether it promotes harm minimisation. Many information leaflets and booklets for gamblers have been produced and made available in venues, but very few have been evaluated (Hing, 2004).

Although not explicitly discussed in the Productivity Commission report (1999), nor elsewhere in the literature, there is a tension between independent bodies inquiring into types of gambling information and options for consumers, and the industry. Objections or counter-arguments by the gambling industries have sometimes been seen as sinister (Costello & Millar, 2000), but it appears that the very nature of harm minimisation, its pragmatic honesty if you will, is in opposition to the whole ethos and attraction of gambling as entertainment. Gambling promotions are not necessarily dishonest, given they stress phantasy, escape and dreams, although it can be argued they come previously close to being misleading on occasions when seeming to overstate the likelihood of winning. There is a fundamental clash of values between on the one hand the attraction of gambling, how it is advertised, and even how some products are sold (see p. 118), and on the other hand all proactive harm prevention strategies, whether viewed through the lens of harm minimisation, "responsible gambling" or consumer protection.

Preventing Problem Gamblers from Further Harm

The training of gambling industry staff, at all levels, was probably pioneered by Harrahs who were among the first to report on the issue of problem gambling amongst industry staff members (Eadington, 1996). Most large companies require staff to complete courses in "responsible gambling" provided by independent educational establishments: courses that work to a specified curriculum and result in a diploma or award. Training includes information about pathological/problem gambling, its incidence and its characteristics, the types of help available, the operation of voluntary self-exclusion programmes, and their role in assisting players who may admit to having problems arising from their gambling.

These latter themes relate to the second broad set of "responsible gambling" strategies designed *to protect the problem player from further excessive gambling*. Internet sites of leading casino companies indicate their priorities in this respect:

- *" . . . is committed to promoting responsible behaviour amongst its guests . . . "*
- *" . . . we do not want compulsive gamblers in our casinos"* (http://www. harrahs.com/about_us/responsible_gaming/ 2002).

Concerns about future litigation drive the latter objective, as it is illegal to knowingly sell gambling to a pathological gambler. Thus the Australian Gaming Commission (an industry lobby group) was involved in facilitating the discussion between international experts on problem gambling, focusing on whether the individual problem gambler could be detected while in the venue. There was general agreement that although a variety of observations could improve the likelihood of estimating that a particular consumer was a problem gambler, sure identification was not possible (Allcock, 2002; Dickerson, 2003b).

Self-exclusion programmes, originally developed by casinos to exclude identified criminals, cheats and even skilled card-counters, today are a key component in "responsible gambling" strategies designed to ensure that identified problem gamblers are not encouraged to enter venues. Although the systems and processes differ from jurisdiction to jurisdiction (Gambling Research Panel

(GPR), 2003a), the fundamental structure is that the self-identified problem gambler makes a binding and enforceable agreement to not enter a casino or set of gaming venues for an agreed period of time, typically at least 1 year. The casino, or gaming industry group if several venues are involved, undertake to "enforce" this ban primarily by detecting such individuals at the venue entrance by a variety of means ranging from the use of photographs to detailed personal identification in the Netherlands (Nowatzki & Williams, 2002). There have been no published accounts of research designed to establish the efficacy of this harm minimisation strategy: most systems have only input data describing the characteristics of the participants rather than the outcome of the self-exclusion. Ladouceur et al. (2000) reported on 220 self-excluders from the Quebec casino: 62% were male, 71% had gambling debts and almost all scored in the pathological gambler range on the South Oaks Gambling Screen (SOGS, Lesieur & Blume, 1987). Two-thirds of a small subgroup that returned to renew their exclusion reported that they had not entered the casino during the initial period of exclusion.

Overall only a very small proportion of problem gamblers use self-exclusion programmes, in Australia approximately 3% of the estimated prevalence (GPR, 2003b) and possibly fewer in Canada, 0.4–1.5% (Nowatzki & Williams, 2002), but the case can be made that such systems have a part to play in the overall group of harm minimisation strategies, perhaps acceptable as a first step in seeking help (Ladouceur et al., 2000) and as one component in a range of supporting professional services. In the absence of regulatory sanctions, self-exclusion involving many venues in the same locality is notoriously difficult to reliably sustain.

Rendering the Process of Gambling Safer for all Consumers

The third set of harm minimisation strategies focused on the possibility of making safer the actual process of continuous forms of gambling. From the frame of reference of mental disorder, it is logical to hypothesise that there may be aspects of the gambling process that is uniquely able to satisfy the needs of the pathological gambler. More generally, the argument has taken the form that the process of gambling as exemplified by the EGM, off-course betting and casino table games is a conditioning process leading to impaired control in regular players, a type of impairment qualitatively different from that experienced by pathological gamblers, but still generating excessive gambling (Blaszczynski & Nower, 2002). The challenge has been to discover which particular structural characteristic of the various gambling formats (e.g. Griffiths, 1993a), if removed or changed, will reduce this addictive effect without spoiling the enjoyment of the majority of ordinary gamblers.

The first illustration of this approach arose in the Netherlands, the "14 Points" from the Nijpels Committee. Peter Reimers from Jellinek Consultancy (Netherlands) outlined the 14 points in his presentation "The Economic and Social Impacts of Gambling in Europe" at the National Association for Gambling Studies conference in Melbourne, November 1997. The 14 suggested changes to EGM operation (e.g. slower reel speed, automatic pay-out, 15 second freeze) represented a harm minimisation strategy designed to prevent the pathological player continuing to gamble excessively. The 14 points were based on anecdotal evidence from problem gamblers in Holland and no empirical evidence or theoretical reasoning was given in support of them other than the type of speculations about structural effects listed by Griffiths (1993a). In addition, there was no understanding of the potential impact on non-problem players. Nonetheless, the changes were legislated and introduced.

The first published field study examining the effects of changing structural characteristics of EGMs on player behaviours and attitudes was completed by Alex Blaszczynski and colleagues with the support of the NSW Government and financed by a representative group of the gaming industry (Blaszczynski et al., 2001). This major project had the strengths of focusing on real players in actual gaming venues, but also the weaknesses of a field study driven by pragmatic concerns rather than theoretical questions. The selection of the structural characteristics was determined by the government harm minimisation policy which had identified three strategies:

1. the removal of high denomination note acceptors,
2. slowing reel spin plus pause to ensure games were no faster than every 5 seconds,
3. reducing the maximum stake per game from $10 to $1.

The Gaming Industry Operators (GIO) approached the University of Sydney Gambling Research Unit offering funding for an independent evaluation of these proposed changes. The research was managed by the University on the basis of a contract that guaranteed the open publication of the results, included independent ethics evaluation and ensured the independence of the actual research team. There was considerable additional support from the industry at all levels from the design of the machine changes, the setting-up of the venues selected for the research, and the provision of player tracking data. As noted earlier, this kind of realistic gambling research can only be conducted with the full collaboration of the industry, and thus requires safeguards (as appears to have existed in this case) to ensure the integrity of such projects is not compromised.

The dependent variables selected to evaluate the changes were player satisfaction and gaming behaviour, the latter either observed in the field by research assistants or tracked via the players' membership card inserted in the machine (only those giving informed permission for their data to be released were included). The key independent variable was the classification of the players into problem and non-problem players using the SOGS (Lesieur & Blume, 1987). Unfortunately the version of the SOGS used was the original lifetime version so there was no certainty that "problem gamblers" had experienced difficulties during the past 12 months. In addition, there was no assessment of the player's current level of involvement in gambling. Consequently, the problem–non-problem gambler comparisons were confounded; differences between the groups could have arisen from different proportions of regular gamblers as opposed to infrequent players. (This point is compounded by the comment in the report that in hotel venues few regular gamblers agreed to participate in the research.)

The machine modifications were contained in a standard popular machine and all possible permutations of the changes were studied to ensure that the effects of all three variables could be separately evaluated. The modified machines were "paired" with "normal" machines and clearly identified in roped off areas in the hotel and club venues for the periods of the research. Convenience recruitment was conducted by the research assistants, and players who participated were required to play a minimum of 20 games on modified and comparison machines.

The strongest measured effect was that all three changes resulted in a significantly lower player expenditure on the modified machines; in particular, limiting the note acceptor to $20 reduced the take by 42%. Enjoyment ratings were most reduced for all players by the slowing of the reel spin. Slowing the game playtime was also found to result in longer sessions of play for some problem gamblers. The impact of reducing the maximum stake per game to $1 was complex, generally reducing play duration but with improved satisfaction ratings by problem players (but only for those in hotels, not in the club venues). It is not possible to interpret the meaning of these results for stake size, as the report fails to specify how the limit of $1 was "enforced". It will be recalled from Chapter 3 that contemporary EGMs in NSW have three key cost factors: the denomination of the machine, the number of winning lines and the bet multiplication. Depending on which one(s) was altered, a different result might be predicted (Haw, 2000).

One other major concern about this field study was that the machine changes were studied over a very short period of a few weeks with players typically playing modified machines just the once, and for a few minutes only. If, as reviewed and shown in various studies, regular players have many hours of conditioning experience that alters their experience and behaviours during the gaming process compared with infrequent players, then studies that evaluate changes to EGM structural characteristics need to not just evaluate the initial response patterns of players but also to study how players learn during repeated experience of the structural changes. It seems quite possible that regular players (including problem players) may show the largest initial disruption of their usual pattern of play and subsequently adapt to the repeated use of the "new" machine, thereby returning to their original style of play.

An independent evaluation of the project report (Tse et al., 2003), notwithstanding their failure to note the confounding of the independent variables of problem and regular gambling, reached a generally favourable impression of the project, suggesting that reducing the stake per game was a potential harm reduction measure meriting further evaluation. The project perhaps both encourages further investigation of the impact of altering machine characteristics whilst also providing salutary lessons of fundamental confounders to be avoided.

A laboratory study has also explored the harm minimisation potential of changes to the structural characteristics of EGMs (Loba et al., 2001). The changes included the provision of a cash counter recording expenditure, another game that did not have the usual touch screen facility enabling the player to stop a selected spinning wheel, and "sensory" changes which unfortunately confounded two changes, slowing the game speed and removing the sound effects. This latter change had the most robust impact, especially on the players scoring in the pathological gambler category, reducing all aspects of their enjoyment. The relevance of this to the real world of gaming venues is not known, as the 60 participants were given cash with which to gamble and all the dependent variables were measured by subjective ratings rather than actual gambling behaviour.

Another laboratory study in Canada examined the impact of breaks in EGM play, either with or without on-screen text messages that reminded the player that all outcomes were chance determined, etc. (Ladouceur & Sevigny, 2003). From a cognitive perspective the authors predicted the greater efficacy of text messages in reducing persistence, but found both conditions had a similar effect compared with a standard game without breaks. Whether this is further evidence for the impact of slowing the EGM (i.e. a more behavioural than cognitive intervention) is doubtful, as the participants were provided with their gambling money. Although the sequence of wins and losses was controlled for all groups, whether the hit rate and other key aspects of the EGMs were similar to the machines that participants played in real venues was not specified.

Dickerson (1999) canvassed the possibility that rather than removing the addictive component from the EGM, it might be preferable to introduce interactive player features that would ensure that, regardless of the duration of a session, the player was making an informed choice to continue to gamble. The hypothetical scenarios were predicated on the assumption that player tracking was operating; that is, the EGM "knew" the player and could check after so many games whether a player knew how long they had played, how much they lost/spent, etc., and whether they wished to continue. Schellinck & Schrans (2002) reported on the first attempt to examine the effect of such messages on player behaviour in real venues. The responsible gaming features introduced by the Nova Scotia Gaming Corporation had the objective of enabling players to manage their time and money expenditure. The features consisted of on-screen clocks, a cash summary of gaming, pop-up reminders of duration of continuous gaming, and enforced cash-out at 150 min after a 5 min prior warning. Unfortunately, other changes to machines over-lapped the evaluation of these features, with new machines faster and with note-acceptors! A number of positive player responses were recorded in the research, although changes to actual gaming behaviour in terms of session length were very small (Schellinck & Schrans, 2002). It must be noted that the features in this project could not be "addressed" to a particular player as there was no tracking: in other words, pop-up notices could be avoided by a player moving to a new machine or cashing out and continuing on the same machine. Nonetheless, this project remains only the second naturalistic study of EGM changes and, more importantly, is part of an ongoing process of harm minimisation evaluation in Nova Scotia.

Despite the methodological concerns about the field studies conducted in Sydney and Nova Scotia, both were very challenging projects and represent the future direction for research into harm minimisation. The former study is specifically endorsed as an example of a collaborative, "science-based approach" in a recent position paper, "the Reno Model" on "responsible gambling"/harm minimisation (Blaszczynski et al., 2004). Before discussing the Reno Model the underlying assumptions of the strategy of "removing" the addictive component of the EGM needs to be challenged.

The best starting point is the Productivity Commission (1999) results confirming the very large increase in "at risk" gamblers associated with regular gambling on continuous forms. As reviewed earlier, roughly the same increase is shown for regular players who prefer EGMs, off-course betting and casino table games, and our own limited work generalised the findings about impaired control of regular EGM players to off-course betting (O'Connor & Dickerson,

2003). In a recent review of the literature Dowling et al. (2005) came to a similar conclusion noting that there is no justification for calling EGMs the "crack-cocaine of gambling": all continuous forms of gambling showing a similar pattern of risk for regular gamblers. Despite reaching this conclusion Dowling et al. (2005) then revisit the speculative work of Griffiths (1993a) and reaffirm the value of examining in isolation the structural characteristics of EGMs to identify those that are the most addictive! In other words, they are ignoring the existing structural evidence that other forms of continuous gambling are equally addictive.

It makes more logical sense, rather than limiting the discussion to EGM structural characteristics, to make the general case that the structural characteristics of *continuous forms* of gambling cause impaired control in regular gamblers, impaired control that may eventuate in harmful impacts. Framed in this way, the question of one structural aspect, for example, the speed of the cycle of stake, play and determination, can be revisited. In the broad context of continuous forms of gambling, it is no longer possible to suggest a particular speed/time that may uniquely contribute to the development of impaired control. The duration of the cycle varies from the 3.5 s on some EGMs to several minutes in off-course betting. The question of slowing the EGM to the pace of off-course betting might appear frivolous, but in a sense it has already been evaluated by the industry. Such slow "EGMs" can still be attractive to players provided a simulated race, even one involving small metal figures on a track, is added (such a machine can be found at the Adelaide casino). The stimulus changes throughout the temporal sequence of the different forms are so very different it is difficult to specify just the crucial factors, other than those central to gambling per se, that is, money is repeatedly staked on uncertain outcomes.

Arguments in support of the relevance of the specific structural changes investigated in the laboratory (Loba et al., 2001), and in the field (Blaszczynski et al., 2001), can only be made by ignoring the structural characteristics of other, equally "addictive" forms of continuous gambling. Thus the examination of the structural characteristics of EGMs, taken in isolation (e.g. Griffiths, 1993a), is misleading when the goal is to understand the origins of impaired control of gambling. A visit to the art department of a well-known EGM manufacturer would have been a salutary experience for anyone wanting to select the most "addictive" aspect of the machine: at one time the walls were covered with sets of artwork from EGM display panels of machines that had failed to be popular with gamblers. *Apart from the artwork, these failures were identical in every respect to existing, successful, machines.*

Impaired Control of Regular Gamblers: A Social and Consumer Protection Issue

If the logical and conceptual basis for changing EGM structural characteristics has been flawed, it nonetheless remains a startling change in policy direction for governments to even consider such a strategy given the revenue implications of disrupting such a popular form of gambling. In Australia the most influential issues have been the estimate that a third of all gambling expenditure/losses (and therefore one-third of the revenue) have come from problem gamblers, and that the majority of clients attending problem gambling services were regular EGM players (Productivity Commission, 1999). This context represents a significant social issue, one that the data on impaired control and its empirical modelling suggests cannot be adequately addressed via any of the "lenses" available under the public health conceptualisation of harm minimisation (Korn et al., 2003; Blaszczynski et al., 2004).

It is helpful to start this discussion by describing what the regular EGM player is doing when gambling. If one takes at random a moment 30 min into a session of play on an EGM by a regular player, the average rate of play would be 13 games per minute and in NSW the maximum stake would be $10 per game. In other words, at this almost halfway stage of a session (in NSW regular players, on average, play for 842 games in a session, range 14–2784: tracking data analysed by Haw, 2000) the player has been offered and purchased a total of 390 games for each of which the possible outcomes ranged from a loss of $10 to a win of $100,000 for a linked machine ($10,000 for a stand-alone machine).

Here we see the individual regular player dealing with a repeated set of purchases where the purchase point of each game is embedded in a rapid sequence of complex winning and losing outcomes. The contemporary language preferred by the industry is that they are providing an entertainment product. No other product that is sold in an automated, unlimited quantity at such a speed comes to mind. Although the per-game cost (on average 40 cents for regular players) appears trivial, the per annum spend of regular players totals about $8000, a major "purchase" for the average wage earner.

On the face of it, these rapid transactions between the player (the consumer) and the provider (the EGM) seem to be contrary to principles of consumer rights. In the process of buying several hundred games, is the choice still an informed choice? Is an awareness of their individual circumstances retained? Is the decision process cool, rational and calm? There is certainly no cooling-off period.

If one now adds the evidence of impaired control, when regular players are sampled (several independent samples) and asked about their experience of controlling their gambling, it is *rare* for a player not to have experienced some, however mild, form of impaired control (15% or less score at the bottom of the range on the Scale of Gambling Choices (SGC)). Forty-three per cent sometimes, often or always experience "an irresistible urge to continue a session of gambling" (O'Connor & Dickerson, 2003).

Given the preferred description of the nature of impaired self-control being an experience common to all human behaviours, rather than being specific to addictive behaviours (Chapter 8, p. 148), then it might said to be common to consumers while shopping to spend more than planned, to experience an urge to spend more, etc. This seems likely to be so, particularly in the context of soaring personal debt in Australia. Nonetheless the occurrence of clinical cases of uncontrolled shopping are relatively rare, and it seems likely that the experience of failing to stick to a budget does not commonly cause significant harm. In contrast, the reports of impaired control among regular EGM players is strongly and positively correlated with significant harmful impacts that can be pervasive and destructive in the gambler's life.

If one now adds the evidence of the factors that contribute to impaired control . . . that is, from the modelling it was shown that greater impaired control arose for players who play more frequently and for longer and show greater emotional reactions to the process of purchasing (i.e. gambling) enhanced, particularly in women by any prior level of non-clinical levels of negative mood, and in men, by hazardous levels of alcohol consumption and impulsivity.

It would appear that the research sequence reported in this monograph has shown the obvious: this is the description of a normal human response to several hours a week consuming an extremely attractive entertainment product that, because of its historical origins as an apparently innocuous mechanical gambling device, is now permitted to be sold as an automated, rapid and emotionally distracting product of unlimited sequences in venues specially designed to heighten the focus on gambling and that are also licensed for the sale and consumption of alcohol. This is not a criticism of the gaming industry or machine manufacturers; it merely illustrates how the analysis of the situation of problem gambling seems trapped by history, both by:

• The evolution of the EGM from slower more humble origins. (The formula for expected loss per hour from the Productivity Commission (1999) shows that the maximum loss per hour has risen from $5.40 in 1956 to $486 in the mid-1990s.)

- The shedding of the language of gambling in policy development and thereby also some of the guiding principles that safeguarded the gambler such as avoiding stimulating demand, casino membership rules, etc.
- The research assumption that impaired control of gambling was the central feature of a mental disorder, pathological gambling, experienced by a small proportion of the population.

If the "Reno Model" succeeds in its goal of influencing the future direction of research and harm minimisation policy in gambling, it is unfortunate that one of its foundations, a classification of gamblers in terms of risk of harm, makes unreferenced assumptions that contradict findings in the literature. *"Players at medium to high risk typically are regular gamblers and at times gamble more than intended; however, their gambling pattern remains in the no harm spectrum."* (p. 13) Much earlier reviews have recorded how common the experience of impaired control is amongst regular gamblers (e.g. Corless & Dickerson, 1989), and as detailed above recent research in both Nova Scotia and Australia has confirmed this for EGM regular players in particular. Detailed databases from two independent research groups (i.e. Schellinck and Schrans in Nova Scotia and Dickerson and colleagues in NSW) have consistently shown that it is *rare* for regular EGM players *not to experience some level of impaired control* over time and money expenditure. This is entirely compatible with the Productivity Commission (1999) finding that one of every five regular players was at risk of significant harmful impacts arising from their gambling. Nonetheless, the Reno model affirms, *"Finally, in the gambling-related harm cell are the minority of players who have developed more serious problems with their gambling, that is, apparent loss of control over time and money spent gambling."* (p. 13) It is possible that the authors are referring to a different conceptualisation of "loss of control" akin to the central tenet of illness, or disease, models of alcohol and drug addiction, one qualitatively different from notions of *impaired*-control residing on a continuum, as a matter of degree (as defined and measured in this monograph), but they do not say this.

The "responsible gambling" approach of the Reno Model to the situation of the regular EGM player identified above is: *"Any 'responsible gambling' program rests upon two fundamental principles: (1) the ultimate decision to gamble resides with the individual and represents a choice, and (2) to properly make this decision, individuals must have the opportunity to be informed. Within the context of civil liberties, external organizations cannot remove an individual's right to make decisions."* (p. 318) The authors argue that the former precludes the imposition of, for example, time limits to gambling duration and the latter, informed choice, is to be supported by information in the form of pamphlets and accurate advertising. The authors seem unsure whether this will be effective but offer no solution: "*Providing information about probabilities and payouts may not be sufficient. Evidence from the research on the effectiveness of primary prevention in the field of substance abuse indicates that increasing knowledge and awareness is insufficient to change behaviour unless values, attitudes and belief structures influencing behaviour are also modified.*" (p. 319) (*Note*: Four different types of information pamphlets have been available in all NSW venues for some years and were available and visible in displays during recruitment for the studies reported in this monograph.)

Thus under the Reno Model, the "responsible gambling" buck is passed back to the regular player. One could hypothesise that it would take a very unusual, highly motivated individual with considerable training to be able to maintain control over the rapid sequence of purchasing decisions described above for the EGM, and this is exactly what the literature shows for successful professional gamblers (Allcock & Dickerson, 1986), except they of course, never use EGMs. Such players approach gambling with a work ethic, devoting many hours daily to learning skills, mastering new information in order to make rational decisions, well aware of potential hazards of emotional involvement and loss of control.

Contemporary gambling, particularly the EGM, is marketed as a leisure and entertainment product. Therefore, the possibility that "responsible gambling" strategies might seek to ensure that all regular players gamble "like" professional gamblers is open to speculation, but is essentially foolish. It remains possible that the introduction of information features on EGMs that require responses from the player (i.e. a player identified by a tracking system) may ensure that she/he is continuing to make free and informed choices. Whether this can be achieved without disrupting the enjoyment of all players is uncertain, and a successful solution will take significant research time, funding and effort.

The application of the "lenses" of the public health model to the harmful impacts of gambling fails to make a vital distinction between gambling and, for example, the consumption of alcohol. In alcohol consumption, the harm arises from the process of ingesting the alcohol and doing so to excess (Pols & Hawks, 1991), in gambling it arises from the process of purchasing itself, especially continuous forms on a regular basis.

The dilemma posed by the commonly experienced impaired control of regular EGM players is not adequately resolved by the lenses provided under the public health model of harm minimisation. The problem has all the appearance of a social and consumer issue (Dickerson, 2003b; IPART, 2004). Some of the most relevant comments to such an issue are to be found in one of the few scholarly appraisals of the ethics of contemporary gambling (Black & Ramsay, 2003). Arguing from a moral realist base, the authors establish that gambling is not wrong per se and develop generic principles that gamblers and gambling providers should follow in order to act ethically. In the social context of the known severe harmful impacts of gambling, and the portrayal by some that the gambling industry exploits human weakness, " The only genuine defence to that portrayal is for the industry to respect human freedom, . . . that impairment of consumer freedom is never intentionally exploited, and that gamblers are helped to maintain self-control throughout their wager . . . should operate gambling activities in a way that avoids taking advantage of people when their self-control is impaired." (pp. 210–211) Does this lead to the conclusion that the contemporary EGM is an unethical method of providing gambling to the regular player?

One method of defending the freedom of choice and informed choice of the regular EGM player already exists in "pre-commitment", which was canvassed among the many harm minimisation strategies by the Productivity Commission (1999) and linked to this specific context by Dickerson (2003b). Pre-commitment involves a player specifying time and/or monetary limits to a session of gambling before purchasing the first game (placing the first bet) in a place away from the influences of the gaming floor. In order to adequately address the aspect of impaired control that leads to the return to a venue to start another session of gambling, such self-imposed limits would have to be binding for a minimum period of at least 24 hours. Otherwise it would be no different from the current situation where a player may purchase a carton of tokens and then return for more. As the gambling industry plans the change to cashless systems, especially for EGMs, there already exist a variety of smartcard and web-based systems that enable all players to be covered by this method of consumer protection.

Under such a system the purchase point has been removed from the emotionally engaging, rapid sequence of gaming and significant purchasing decisions can be made away from the gaming floor, in private, advised by a variety of pamphlets (and even computer simulations) calculating the likely rate of expenditure (losses) for the individuals preferred pattern of staking. From both the perspective of the player and the provider under such a system of consumer protection, the conflicting goals of each are resolved: the former is free to "lose control" as part of the gambling experience and the latter to develop venue themes that enhance the entertainment of the player regardless of its impact on player self-control. Such systems also have the capacity to effectively support self-exclusion and a range of "responsible gambling" strategies while at the same time maintaining the anonymity of the player. They would also virtually eliminate underage gambling on whatever gambling products were covered by such a system.

Consumer protection measures of this nature do not replace the harm minimisation strategies described as "responsible gambling" they enable them to make sense, to make reasonable, mutually appropriate demands on both the provider and the gambler. Under such systems gamblers may choose to set limits that result in excessive expenditure and harmful impacts to themselves and those around them just as any person with a credit card may choose to spend beyond their means. This sort of choice by gamblers would indeed be *"one of deciding not to exercise control"* (Edwards & Gross, 1976, p. 1060). However, the excessive expenditure resulting from those levels of impaired control typically experienced during a session of gambling, that are genuinely beyond the ability of the person to control at that moment in time would be prevented.

In our opinion there has been a failure in consumer protection not to safeguard the rights of gamblers and the processes of selling/providing continuous forms of gambling need to be modified to maintain the same standards expected for any other entertainment product. This failure is a social issue and one that may gain sufficient momentum to influence a shift in policy given the recent involvement of Ralph Nader (Insight Conference, Nova Scotia Gaming Foundation, October 2004). He drew parallels with his earliest successful consumer rights projects involving automobiles; summarizing these as a shift in responsibility for the harm caused by crashes *from the driver to the industry* and the latter's subsequent evolution of automobile safety features. How could the responsible driver protect themselves and their passengers when no seat belts were fitted? The current emphasis of the gambling industry, government and problem gambling experts enshrined in "responsible gambling" is also on the "driver", the gambler, who must learn to exercise self-control in the venue while actually gambling. Ralph Nader endorsed the need for and the advantages of technological "pre-crash" interventions such as pre-commitment systems that safeguard the gambler.

Whether such changes also result in harm minimisation is a separate issue. It seems possible and even likely that adequate consumer protection will also reduce the harm from gambling but such changes to continuous forms of gambling should not wait on evidence that they do so. One province in Canada seems likely to act to better defend consumer rights introducing a system whereby all EGMs are operated by a personal player card which is only activated when a limit (i.e. of expenditure of time of money per session, per week) has been specified. At the very least it is important that the public debate in jurisdictions that are considering the transition to convenience access to EGMs (and other forms of continuous gambling) should include information about the availability of such consumer protection systems; systems that leave the gaming process intact but safeguard the purchasing decisions of the gambler.

7

A Case Study of "Responsible Gambling" Strategies within a Single Jurisdiction: Victoria, Australia

The Introduction of Gaming Machines

In this chapter the "case" of the State of Victoria in Australia is presented: the decade from 1992 onwards when first electronic gaming machines (EGMs) and then a casino were made legally available, the population changes in the gambling attitudes and behaviours, the economic impacts and the complex set of social policies that were developed to assess, manage and prevent the harmful impacts arising from gambling. This "case" is intended neither as a moral argument nor a salutary tale, merely a description of a relatively small jurisdiction (3.6 million aged 15 years and older; ABS, 2003 census data) reacting politically and socially to the introduction of 30,000 EGMs. In the same period, of all the states and territories in Australia in which occurred similar changes in the availability of EGMs, the response of Victoria has been the most comprehensive, arguably setting International benchmarks in research, service delivery and harm minimisation (note possible conflict of interest for MD; see declaration at Preface).

The "snapshot" of Victoria provided by the 2001 census data (ABS, 2003) locates about one quarter of the Australian population in this state on the south-eastern corner of the continent. The 0.5% of the 4.6 million is of Indigenous origin, 52% are married (or de facto), 71% Australian born and over 80% dwell in urban settings. The linguistic mix provides some indication of the cultural diversity: English is the language spoken at home for 75%, but 3.2% speak Italian, 2.7% Greek and 2.5% Chinese, indicating the strong theme of cultural diversity. The median household size is 2.6 persons, median income A\$800–999 per week, the median age is 35 years, 6.8% are unemployed and two-thirds go to work by car.

The introduction of EGMs was delayed by about a decade by an inquiry (Wilcox, 1983) that detailed the inadequacies of gaming policy and regulation in the neighbouring state of New South Wales (NSW), and noting the potential

124

for increased criminal activity, recommended against the introduction of "poker machines" as they were called, to Victoria. Nonetheless, the role of the "neighbour" was eventually the determining factor in the introduction of EGMs in 1992. In common with the contemporary experience in the USA where native Indian territories have a casino, the border with NSW was marked by the presence of very large social clubs (with many poker machines), with large parking areas for coaches. There was in economic terms considerable "leakage" of potential gambling revenue out of Victoria as people travelled from all over the state to spend the day gaming (playing EGMs) in NSW.

After a brief experiment with a cashless form of new machine, the *Gaming Machine Control Act 1991* provided for two operators (Tattersall's and the Totalisator Agency Board (TAB), renamed Tabcorp after privatisation in 1994) to purchase and install EGMs in clubs and hotels and to operate a centralised monitoring system (CMS). In what has been described as a highly interventionist government approach (VCGA, 1999), the CMS was a critical factor in allowing the legalisation of EGMs. The system enabled the real-time monitoring of all machines 24 hours a day, recording all games played, the amount wagered, prizes paid and the cash retained. This information provided security, aiding the operators in marketing decisions, and accessed by government regulators for financial control and auditing.

On the 16th July 1992, EGMs at two venues in Melbourne began operations. In 1994 the Melbourne "Crown Casino" opened in temporary premises with 130 gaming tables and 1200 EGMs. Originally a state-wide cap of 45,000 machines was envisaged but in 1995 this was revised to 30,000, pending the outcomes of independent research into the social and economic impacts. This limit has been reached and still prevails, with the maximum of 2500 in the casino included in the total, giving a machine density of about one per 120 adults (about a third of the density in NSW which currently has 100,000 machines for a slightly larger population).

Just 4 years later, by 1998, expenditure on EGMs accounted for about 60% of per capita gambling expenditure, rising to 90% within the decade when added to the expenditure at the casino. In the same period, gambling taxation as a percentage of total Victorian state government taxation recorded a rise of 5% to around 15% that was almost entirely attributable to EGMs.

The popularity of EGM play was rapidly established as shown in Figure 7.1 and has remained fairly stable until the most recent survey completed in 2003 (GRP, 2004). It has remained the third most popular form of gambling after lotteries and instant (scratch) lotteries. Regular weekly or more frequent EGM players are less prevalent than in NSW (3% compared to 10%). This difference

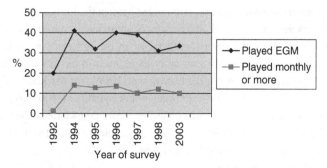

Figure 7.1. Percentage of the population of Victoria (Australia) who played EGMs during the past 12 months (adapted from Dickerson, 2003a).

has been attributed to lower machine density (GRP, 2004), but may also be because of the different venues preferred by the majority of regular players in each state; in Victoria hotels and bars are preferred whereas in NSW the preferred venue is the registered club, many of which are the size of casinos with a wide range of entertainments and restaurants, thereby attracting a demographically much broader and larger patronage.

Almost half the regular EGM players have sessions longer than 90 min, 36% spend more than planned (sometimes, often or always) compared with 3.4% of infrequent gamblers and 57% travel less than 5 km from home to their preferred venue (GRP, 2004). Typically, the regular EGM player also participates in lotteries and instant lotteries and places bets occasionally on major race meetings, such as the Melbourne Cup. The per capita expenditure on gambling in Victoria has risen to about $1000 (3.5% of Household Disposable Income) (Tasmanian Gaming Commission, 2004), two-thirds of which is spent on EGM play.

Thus EGMs "arrived" in Victoria and became established as the most popular form of continuous gambling. Over the same period there was a similar picture of evolution in several other states in Australia, but in Victoria the response to dealing with all aspects of the harmful impacts arising from the new EGM gambling and all other forms was the most comprehensive. Two key reasons for this might be, first that the Premier at the time was perceived as being close to key stakeholders developing the casino and operating the EGMs and therefore as the party in power the Liberals were very keen to take the moral high ground in the provision of all possible services for problem gamblers. Secondly, just as specified in the Gaming Machine Control Act, 8.3% of the daily cash flow from the EGMs in hotels began to stream into the Public Account of the Community Support Fund. Coincidentally there were two very competent and creative public servants in the Department of Human Services (DHS) who put forward a proposal for funding an integrated problem gambling services strategy.

The Victorian Problem Gambling Services Strategy

The first triennial grant provided by the Community Support Fund lead to the implementation of the following:

- Problem gambling counselling services, integrated with financial counselling.
- A Gambler's Help Line, free, 24-h telephone counselling and referrals (originally called G-Line).
- Gambling liaison and community education officers in each DHS region.
- Community education and media awareness campaigns.
- A liaison group chaired by the DHS and with representatives from all sectors, industry, community and counselling agencies.
- A research programme focussing on problem gambling, its causes and management (complimenting the research programme of the Victorian Casino and Gaming Authority (VCGA) which funded projects examining the economic and social impacts of gambling, until both research programmes were amalgamated under the Gambling Research Panel (GRP) in 2001).

All of the individual themes listed above can be found in the policy responses to problem gambling in many other jurisdictions internationally, but the breadth of content, and above all, the integration of all these components may be claimed to be unique in Victoria. This integration is best illustrated by the way in which the advertising campaigns designed to heighten community awareness about the harmful impacts of gambling evolved over a 5-year period into a fully fledged health promotion strategy.

Problem Gambling Community Education Campaigns

Launched in November 1995, the first campaign consisted of three key stages:

1. The five weeks based around print (newspaper advertisements and billboards) and radio advertisements. The latter were in English, Arabic, Vietnamese, Cantonese and Macedonian.
2. The 14 weeks of television advertising showing a problem gambler's crisis, for example a mother stealing from her own child's piggy bank to support her gambling.
3. Combined radio and TV advertising (Total budget about $2.5 million). The campaign education message was "If you have a problem with gambling

call...." and gave the toll-free Help Line number. This advertising was supported by local, community based work by the liaison officers who were appointed to each of the health areas as part of the staffing of the counselling services for problem gamblers.

In a generally favourable evaluation (Jackson et al., 2000), it was reported that 46% of respondents were able to recall at least one problem gambling related advertisement and there was *a "dramatic and immediate increase in the number of telephone calls ..."* (p. 8) to the Help Line during the second and third phase. The local liaison efforts had resulted in just over half of all gaming venues receiving a visit from a counselling service representative.

The integration of the use of mass media with local education and interventions with collaboration from both the existing services and all components of the gaming industry immediately differentiated this Victorian approach from other gambling education campaigns in the USA, Canada and UK. Most of these have been funded by the industry directly rather than by a government agency, with a limited message and little or no integration with existing services, and targeting the pathological gambler. For example "Gambling should remain a game" Loto-Quebec, Canada.

The Victorian campaign had much more in common with best practice in public health campaigns and this was further developed in the two subsequent campaigns:

- Myths campaign (1998–February 2000), cost about $2 million, "If it's No Longer Fun, Walk Away" was the slogan and "at risk" gamblers were the target. This was not evaluated and was terminated at the change of government in 2000.
- "Think of What You're Really Gambling With" campaign (from November 2000 to 2005), targeting problem and "at risk" gamblers, budget about $16.5 million.

The third and current campaign was based on research and consultation with key stakeholders and was comprehensively designed to contact all those who were affected by problem gambling: dealing with cultural and linguistic factors, age, gender and location within the state boundaries. The two direct services, the telephone line and the counselling services were renamed, "Gambler's Help" and there was:

- a television, radio and print campaign and additional more focussed themes;
- convenience advertising in all venues and *maintained* throughout the whole period of the campaign;

- community information including Self-Help manuals, and local lectures and talks by the liaison officers from the counselling services;
- public relations exercises with the Minister touring regional centres;
- campaigns targeting specific populations, for example posters focussing on aboriginal gambling issues.

This was clearly more than a campaign. It was a communication strategy. Problem gambling was conceptualised along a continuum of harm risk, with the message at each point of risk tailored to meet the potential needs of the individual at that point. The underlying model of attitude and behaviour change adopted was the *"Stages of Behaviour Change"* (Prochaska & DiClemente, 1988) and consumers could identify the potential harms of gambling, self-assess and receive information about the existing services. The first evaluation by market research (Sweeney Research, 2001) confirmed the high levels of community awareness and the increased contacts with both the Help Line and the counselling services especially during periods when the television advertisements were screened.

The Ottawa Charter defines health promotion as "the process of enabling people to increase control over, and to improve, their health" (WHO, 1997). The "Think of What You're Really Gambling With" campaign is appropriately considered as a "health promotion campaign". The following sections that describe some of the specific counselling services and harm minimisation strategies should be seen in this overall context of integration.

Direct Treatment Services

The DHS established counselling services (The *BreakEven* network) throughout the state, integrating the existing regional patterns of delivery of other health and human services with a detailed knowledge provided by the VCGA of the distribution of the new EGMs. Thus more services were planned for areas where machine density was greatest. The services were provided by non-government agencies employing professionally qualified social workers and psychologists who used a wide range of counselling approaches with client problem gamblers. Service delivery was typically from community centres with a variety of "outreach" offices, so that within a few years the number of points at which clients could access services was more than 100. As part of the contractual standard operating procedures all services collected the minimum data set (MDS) describing client characteristics, the services delivered and the outcome. These are analysed annually and published by DHS.

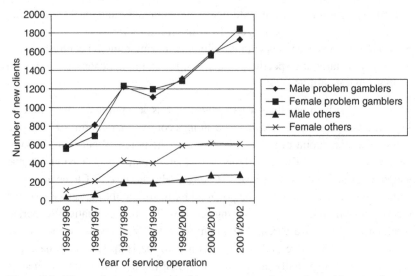

Figure 7.2. The total number of new clients per annum, by gender and by type, for each year of service operation (adapted from Dickerson, 2003a).

Ever since the services began to operate, the number of new clients seeking help from the services has steadily increased (see Figure 7.2). Any person, either directly concerned with their own gambling issues or concerned about those of a relative or friend, may attend for free counselling. The term "problem" gamblers is used as defined in Dickerson et al. (1997) meaning that the person is experiencing harmful impacts arising from their own or another's gambling.

New clients, 4461, registered between 1 July 2001 and 30 June 2002, representing an 18.3% increase for women problem gamblers and 9.4% for men problem gamblers compared with 2000–2001. The "other" new clients comprised mainly the spouse of a gambler or other family members: the service funding permits family members adversely affected by gambling to attend for counselling even if the problem gambler her/himself does not.

Almost all the client problem gamblers reported an inability to control their gambling behaviour and the most common harmful impacts reported were intrapersonal (depressed mood, low self-esteem), relationship and employment issues. The MDS includes the Diagnostic and Statistical Manual of Mental Disorders, 4th edition (DSM-IV) diagnostic criteria – 91% of all problem gamblers reported the use of gambling as a way of escaping, 80% chased their losses and 83% have repeatedly, but unsuccessfully, attempted to control or stop their gambling; 23% of all new client problem gamblers did not satisfy the diagnostic criteria for "pathological gambling" (DSM-IV), but this is no bar to service delivery: the DHS defines its mandate in terms of problem gambling, preventing and ameliorating the harmful impacts of gambling.

The "role" of EGM gambling in the lives of the new clients is very significant and increasing (see Figures 7.3 and 7.4): 96.2% of women and 78.1% of men preferred this form of gambling, playing EGMs in a typical gambling session lasting 3 h, twice a week and spending about $200 each session. Illegal activities to obtain money for gambling were reported by 21% of men and 14% of women problem gamblers. The mean gambling related debt reported by clients was $35,000 for men and $15,000 for women.

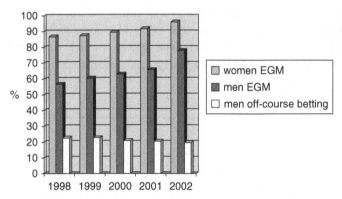

Figure 7.3. Percentage of new client problem gamblers (men and women) by form of gambling and by year of registration (adapted from Dickerson, 2003a). (Note: Off-course betting is very rarely the preferred form of women problem gamblers.)

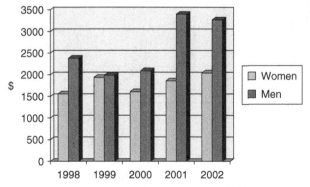

Figure 7.4. Per month expenditure of new client problem gamblers (men and women) for EGM play by year of registration (adapted from Dickerson, 2003a).

Although the data describing problem gamblers attending for counselling are not representative of all gamblers in the community who are experiencing harmful impacts, the indications from the MDS on a variety of measures suggesting that those seeking help since 2000 are reporting more severe problems is potentially very significant. In the context of long-term social planning, it might be argued that a population may slowly learn to gamble on a new product in ways that do not lead to harm, especially if a number of harm minimisation strategies and education programmes are included in a comprehensive set of strategies, as was the case in Victoria. The more recent evidence of increasing severity of problems reported by the new clients (see Figure 7.5) does not support such an argument and is more compatible with the national research finding that, on average, problem gamblers "wait" 7 years before seeking counselling help (Productivity Commission, 1999). In Victoria the first 2 full years of EGM operation were 1993 and 1994. Recent research (O'Connor, 2000; Breen & Zimmerman, 2002) suggesting the rapid development of harmful

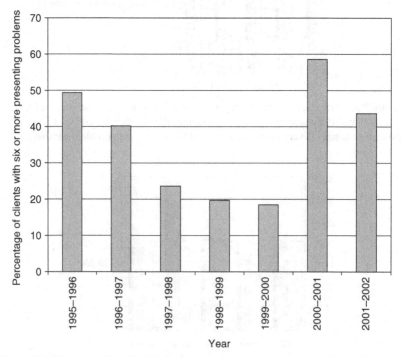

Figure 7.5. The proportion of new clients reporting six or more presenting problems by year of registration (adapted from Dickerson, 2003a).

impacts, contrary to the traditional picture of evolution of pathological gambling over several years (e.g. Custer, 1984), suggests that a jurisdiction, such as Victoria, may not be able to fully appreciate the level of harmful impacts experienced by gamblers until more than 7 years after first introducing the new gambling product.

Gambler's Help Line: Ever since the funding of the state-wide counselling service in 1994, the DHS also funded an independent, 24-h toll-free, anonymous telephone line which provided a crisis and referral service. In the same year (2001–2002) described above in which over 4000 new clients registered for counselling, the Help Line responded to over 16,000 telephone calls relating to gambling issues and over 7000 of these callers were referred to local counselling services.

Clients of the telephone Help Line remain anonymous and cannot at present be tracked to the counselling service, although there are discussions about the use of a unique client number system that would permit a better evaluation of the effectiveness of the integration of the two services. On the available data it appears that three out of every four callers referred to counselling do not act on/take up that referral (Dickerson, 2003a).

Harm Minimisation

From the very beginning of problem gambling service provision in Victoria harm minimisation themes of educating gamblers, minimal interventions, self-assessment and self-help materials were included. The preference for the terms "problem gambler" rather than the mental disorder conceptualisation encouraged a more pragmatic generalisation from existing services for alcohol problems, and the appointment of the liaison officers ensured that a service presence was potentially available in every venue. In addition, the gambling industry either was required by government, or volunteered, to develop other harm minimisation themes.

Prior to the introduction of EGMs, casino inquiries in other states (e.g. *Street Report* to the NSW Government, 1991) had specified that ATMs should be placed away from the gaming floor. This was a regulatory requirement in Victoria ab initio and since then, depending on the government of the day and its policy on responsible gambling, other changes, such as clocks in venues, windows and, most recently, smoke-free gaming, have been required. (The latter resulting in an immediate but possibly short-term fall in gaming expenditure of 20–30%.) At the community level the original state-wide cap on the total number of machines was reduced by a third and is now complemented by the requirement for local social impact studies before changes in machine distribution can be considered.

The gambling industry, despite comprising five disparate groups, the registered clubs, hotels, the two EGM operators and the casino, acted collaboratively to promote responsible gambling. They established and funded a secretariat for the Victorian Gaming Machine Industry (VGMI) and provided two integrated definitions of responsible gambling that were much more specific than any previous industry goals or mission statements worldwide.

"The industry's role is to offer products and services in a way that facilitates customers' ability to engage in responsible gaming"

and

"Responsible gaming is each person exercising a rational and sensible choice based on his or her individual circumstance."

The VGMI provided a complaints procedure for consumers and began the process of setting standards for venues and gaming staff and developing staff training in the responsible provision of gaming. Self-exclusion was also developed collaboratively and in theory offers players the opportunity to self-exclude from all EGM venues state-wide, whether in a hotel, club or casino but in reality, depending still on photographic identification is impossible to maintain.

Once past the irony of placing a service for problem gamblers in a casino complex, the "customer support centre" at Crown Casino in Melbourne can be seen to have broken new ground in the responsible provision of gaming. The office of the centre provides instant access to advice and counselling from psychologists and from trained casino staff who "bridge" the gap from gaming floor to the support centre, responding to calls from staff on duty in the EGM areas or table games who may report players in distress or who are actively seeking help, perhaps wanting to establish a self-exclusion order. The opportunity to arrange the latter in a place of privacy with trained staff within a few moments of making the decision to seek help provides a unique opportunity for self-exclusion to be explained and placed in the context of other potentially relevant interventions; the self-exclusion rate per month has doubled since the opening of the centre. The most recent service currently being evaluated by the casino is a pre-commitment procedure whereby club members may arrange for a specific expenditure limit per day or per week to be recorded on their card so that when entered in EGMs played and the limit is reached a message stream running across the face of the machine advises the player that their limit has been reached. Should the player decide to continue, they can do so as all machines operate to cash entered, the membership coloured light shown by the machine extinguishes (under usual operating this light advises venue staff where casino club members are playing) and the continued play by the member no longer accrues privileges and bonuses.

Research

Two government agencies were originally charged with the conduct of research into the social and economic impacts of the introduction of EGMs and the casino, the VCGA and the DHS. The latter's brief was restricted to the evaluation of harm minimisation and direct services for problem gamblers and their families. In 2000 the research planning and coordination was brought together under a single GRP which consults broadly in the community in the development of a planned programme of research goals which is published at its web site (www.grp.vic.gov.au).

The DHS sequence of studies evaluated the longitudinal impact of its service delivery, established the process of regular annual review of the MDS from service centres, evaluated the most effective form of intervention, and studied the impact of EGMs on women players and the impacts of gambling on children and adolescents. The VCGA complemented this work with a sequence of studies first to define problem gambling and then to develop a new population survey method of measurement (Dickerson et al., 1997; Ben-Tovim et al., 2001).

The recommended definition of problem gambling to be adopted in Victoria was:

" '*Problem gambling' refers to the situation when a person's gambling activity gives rise to harm to the individual player, and/or to his or her family, and may extend into the community.*" (Dickerson et al., 1997, p. 2). A primary concern was to avoid the pitfalls of academic dispute about the causes of problem gambling and to ensure that problem gambling research of the VCGA prioritises the assessment of the extent and degree of the harm per se. The authors also provided an illustration of how a multidisciplinary and multi-method approach could develop a balanced and more complete picture of the level of problem gambling in Victoria, one that collated and interpreted a number of independent data streams, and was sensitive to the assessment of problem gambling in a diversity of contexts.

Subsequently a research team from Flinders University was contracted to develop what was released as the Victorian Gambling Screen: a population screen validated to detect the presence of the harmful impacts of gambling (Ben-Tovim et al., 2001). The screen has since been independently evaluated and also used

concurrently with the South Oaks Gambling Screen and the Canadian Problem
Gambling Index (GRP, 2003c).

Victoria: A Successful Public Health Approach or a Failure of Consumer Protection?

The latest estimates of the prevalence of problem gambling in Victoria remain
at about the 1–2% level depending on the measure used and the criteria adopted
(GRP, 2004). 15–20% of regular consumers of continuous forms of gambling
are "at risk" confirming one of the key empirical foundations of the work
reported in this monograph on impaired control. 84% of problem gamblers
prefer EGM play. Male gamblers are at greater risk but this is a function of
proportionally more males being regular gamblers rather than indicating a
greater propensity for males to become problem gamblers. Regular gamblers
from non-English speaking backgrounds are more likely to be problem gamblers,
confirming the findings of an earlier cultural diversity study of the impacts of
gambling (Thomas et al., 2000), but are less likely to access the services provided.

28.7% of problem gamblers surveyed in 2003 (GRP, 2004) reported that
they had sought professional or personal help with their gambling problems.
This closely matched the estimate in the latest review of the new clients attending
counselling (based on the returns for the year July 2001–June 2002) (Dickerson,
2003a) that the service was reaching about one-third of the most serious "cases"
in the general population. This suggests a high standard of accessibility: the
availability of services is well known; the survey found that less than 2% of the
problem gamblers did not know where to go for help, 75% finding out from television advertising. However the most common reason for help seeking was
financial concerns (95%) and the type of help most commonly sought was financial assistance/material aid (59%). In fact, only 10% of problem gamblers sought
help from the Gambler's Help Line and 6% from the counselling services, compared with 35% who went to Gamblers Anonymous, the self-help voluntary
organisation. Taking the survey findings together with the new client data from
the funded services it is apparent that the prevalence of problem gambling in
Victoria may be closer to the 1999 Productivity Commission estimate of 2.1%,
that is approximately 75,000 adults with significant harmful impacts arising from
their gambling during the last 12 months.

Victoria represents a small jurisdiction that has developed the most complete
public health approach to the harmful impacts of gambling. During the first
5 years the expenditure on services and community awareness/health promotion
campaigns averaged A$12 million per annum (VCGA, 2000), not including

the VCGA research programme. Despite the quality and range of the services provided, and the increasing numbers of new clients attending for help, they appear to attract only a small proportion of those in need. The majority of the population consider gambling to represent a serious social problem (84%), one that has become more serious over the last 3 years (80%) (GRP, 2004). The report in summarising the negative attitudes of the majority of the population concluded that there was a readiness for policy change concerning EGMs. One attitude was the strong endorsement of the principle underlying the pre-commitment systems discussed in the previous Chapter: 81% of gamblers and 90% of non-gamblers supported the statement, "People should be able to limit the amount that they can spend at any one time on poker machines".

The case study of Victoria may therefore be seen both as:

- An example of the public health frame of reference applied to the harmful impacts of gambling, perhaps setting international benchmarks for its integration of the components of a responsible gambling strategy, its health promotion campaigns, as well as for the high levels of consultation with and collaboration of all stakeholders.
- An example of the cost both in terms of dollars and human distress of a failure to correctly link the origins of the harmful impacts of gambling with the nature of the consumer purchasing process in EGM play (and probably other forms of continuous gambling) and to ensure the application of existing standards of consumer protection using available technology.

8
Conclusions

Impaired Self-control of Gambling

In Dickerson & Baron (2000) the suggestion was made that research examining problem gambling might be simplified if the preferred dependent variable was impaired self-control rather than the heterogeneous consequences that comprise the diagnostic criteria of pathological gambling (APA, 1994). The proposal was derived from the arguments of Heather et al. (1993) concerning alcoholism: impaired control as *the* essential construct in the psychological conceptualisation of addiction. Impaired self-control of gambling was defined as an inability to consistently maintain preferred limits to expenditure of time and money on gambling. From the evidence and arguments presented in the previous chapters, the following conclusions may be drawn.

Measurement

The most consistent findings have been demonstrated by the measurement of impaired self-control of gambling: the fundamental work of Kyngdon (2003) providing evidence for a continuous quantitative dimension (from effortless self-control to an inability to impose control over their gambling behaviour), and the use of a traditional psychometric approach (Scale of Gambling Choices (SGC), Baron et al., 1995) in a number of studies demonstrated acceptable reliability, validity and factorial coherence (particularly for the 12-item version: O'Connor & Dickerson, 2003; Kyngdon, 2004).

In several studies of large independent samples of regular gamblers (i.e. gambling sessions once per week or more) impaired self-control of gambling has been shown to be a very common experience (e.g. 43% "sometimes", "often" or "always" experience an irresistible urge to continue a session; O'Connor & Dickerson, 2003). Although only one study involved off-course betting, the majority involving electronic gaming machine (EGM) players, it seems probable that impaired self-control is a common feature of regular consumption of all forms of continuous gambling. Measurement studies involving clinical groups of diagnosed pathological gamblers demonstrated that the impairment of self-control reported by these problem gamblers does not differ uniquely from the reports of regular gamblers: there is evidence for a continuum of experience of impaired self-control with problem gamblers showing higher levels on average than regular gamblers.

Key Psychological Variables

Impaired self-control as measured by the SGC consistently, strongly correlates with measures of the harmful impacts of gambling and pathological gambling (the Victorian Gambling Screen (VGS) in O'Connor et al. (2005) and the South Oaks Gambling Screen (SOGS) in Baron et al. (1995)) and in the modelling work of Maddern (2004) impaired self-control was demonstrated to be a key conceptual theme in both the qualitative and quantitative studies of youth gamblers.

In a large sample of regular EGM players recruited in gaming venues (O'Connor et al., 2005), strength of positive emotion experienced during gaming and current level of involvement in gaming were significant predictors of impaired self-control for both men and women, and remained so prospectively at six-month follow-up, still accounting for almost 25% of the variance. There were significant gender differences with impaired control linked to prior negative mood in women and impulsivity and alcohol consumption in men. The preferred speculative interpretation of these findings was that the impaired self-control of regular gamblers was a function of a conditioning process in which the crucial reinforcement was strong positive emotion, heightened by prior non-clinical levels of negative mood in women and personality differences and alcohol use in men.

It was argued that this conditioning, conceptualised as expectations (e.g. Vogel-Sprott & Fillmore, 1999), gave credence to theoretical accounts of gambling derived from models of human decision-making such as regret theory (Baron, 1994) and subjective expected emotion (SEE) (Mellers et al., 1999) may be able to predict the gambling behaviour of regular, and therefore also, problem gamblers. It was further speculated that this emotional conditioning resulted in the addictive behaviour having innate action precedence, particularly so in environments rich in the cues that are associated with the behaviour.

Cognitions and Chasing

Expectations of winning rather than of positive emotions have featured in cognitive accounts of problem gambling (Ladouceur & Walker, 1996). If conditioning is the primary process "driving" the development of impaired self-control, the role of other more commonly cited cognitive processes such as expectations of winning, beliefs about skill and other illusions of control may provide secondary roles. These cognitions may facilitate impaired self-control, experienced as an "urge" to be expressed behaviourally in further gambling, and provide a post hoc self-explanation of why the player persisted despite such losses and avowals to stick to lower limits.

As suggested in earlier discussions it is possible that the phenomenon of chasing bridges both the primary conditioning process and the secondary cognitive processes. When chasing was defined and measured in terms of subjective feelings, thoughts about raising stakes, persistence and actual chasing behaviour, then chasing was revealed to be highly correlated with impaired self-control (O'Connor & Dickerson, 2003 & 2003a).

In the Present Context:

  I. The feeling of wanting to chase may represent the gambler's awareness of the *impact* of the conditioning process, the increased desirability of gambling.
 II. The cognitions featuring the "strategy" of chasing (e.g. the reasoning that only a big win will redress past losses) facilitating the decision to return to the EGM, the next race broadcast.
III. The post hoc naming of the excessive gambling as "chasing" providing a self-explanation, a justification for what happened.

In such a schema, illusory beliefs about the likelihood of winning and about personal skill, would also act at II and III, further supporting the development of impaired control. Thus, the diversity of cognitive themes around gambling represent the player's "struggle" to both understand and make sense of the emerging impaired control as well as developing beliefs that may either limit or facilitate the level of impairment.

On the Nature of Impaired Self-control of Gambling

When the concept of impaired control was first introduced in the context of alcohol dependence, Edwards & Gross (1976) questioned whether this was truly intermittent loss of self-control or rather *"one of deciding not to exercise control"* (p. 1060). More strongly, Davies (1992) argued, *"... most people who use drugs do so for their own reasons, on purpose, because they like it, and because they find no adequate reason for not doing so;"* (p. xi). If some genuine sense of impaired self-control is axiomatic to psychological conceptualisations of addiction (Heather et al., 1993), these questions, veritable horns of a dilemma, merit consideration in the light of the recent research into gambling, a behaviour that is, in the absence of the physiological properties of a psychoactive agent altering emotions, perceptions and cognitions, a potentially more transparent addictive process.

In the following brief speculative section, different levels of impairment of self-control of gambling are considered in terms of the subjective experience of the gambler and the extent to which it may be said the individual can still choose to stop or continue. It has been assumed that impaired self-control is a common human experience, subjectively similar from behaviour to behaviour (not just evident in drug dependence or "addiction") including gambling, given the essentially non-pathological, normal psychological variables found to give rise to impaired self-control over gambling. As the items from the scales developed by Kyngdon (2003) provided evidence for a quantitative dimension of impairment of self-control, the following discussion is anchored around them:

A. I am free to gamble at my leisure as it does not cause any problems and I never experience any need to control my gambling at all.
B. Although I feel a need to control my gambling it is easily controlled without a conscious effort and it does not cause any problems. (p. 123)

The second statement marks a crucial first step in impairment, a step that anticipates the key themes of temptation–restraint (Maddern's (2004) extension of the work of Collins and colleagues). What has given rise to this awareness of the need to take care? Is it similar to the situation of one caller to the toll-free helpline in Victoria: she had been to play the newly available EGMs and found it so very enjoyable that she wondered to the counsellor, "Was this a cause for concern? Might it get out of control?"

The fact that the first item, autonomy, free from impairment, is apparently integrated with the rest of the scale may have no necessary implications for the underlying psychological processes that lead to impairment, but it is possible that the continuity of the dimension of impairment may mean that the same processes are active but to different degrees at each increasing level of impairment. Where gambling is freely initiated and stopped, the associated feelings may be positive enjoyment but fittingly less salient than the positively valenced feelings associated with other more valued activities such as personal relationships, vocational and family duties. For the caller described above, it may be the unusual saliency of the gambling feelings compared with those associated with other core life activities, which gave rise to that initial feeling that care might need to be exercised with regard to future gambling. (It is possible, but seems unlikely, that she would have bothered to make the call simply on the basis of gambling now being popularly defined as a potential problem in the Australian context.) If repeated experiences of EGM play (or other continuous forms of gambling) increase the saliency of the feelings during play (e.g. Moodie & Finnigan, 2005), and pre-existing mild levels of negative mood enhance the saliency still further, perhaps especially in women (Hills et al., 2001; O'Connor et al., 2005), is this the beginning of impaired self-control? Does the increasing saliency of the positive gambling feelings require increased effort or coping resources to enable the player to select and maintain their preferred level of involvement?

C. I feel a need to control my gambling and whilst it is relatively easy to control ... it does require conscious effort ... does not cause any problems ... do think about cutting back from time to time.

D. Although my gambling is relatively difficult to control, it causes few but only minor problems.

Given that coping resources vary in efficacy, have finite limits for any one individual and may be depleted by other life event demands (Muraven & Baumeister, 2000), then occasions will occur when limits cannot be maintained, when the attraction of the gambling feelings will overwhelm coping strategies and self-control cannot be imposed. Whether this is "genuine" impaired control rather than choosing a preferred option may be examined by considering the activities that comprise a session of gambling. During EGM play itself the speed and simple nature of the response (a button press or touch to a screen) together with the associated emotions suggests that even after a few hours total playing time, play may require no conscious monitoring. Players describe coming to "trust" the machine, not to count payouts, not to check all possible paylines, preferring to become engrossed in each moment, enjoying playing repeated games. Such "unconscious" gambling may suggest automata and thereby "genuine" loss of self-control at those moments, but this is not necessarily so.

First, in order to be consistent with our assumption that each point on the scale of impairment is subject to the same psychological processes, the autonomous, self-controlled player may also experience "unconscious" gambling moments, becoming so engrossed in enjoying the action that wider awareness is greatly diminished, perhaps even absent. This gambling experience may be similar to moments of focused pleasure that occur in a variety of activities, and that for example may be specifically sought in sexual behaviour. However, such concentration does imply impairment of self-control because during those periods there is diminished self-awareness of broader contextual cues. Regular gamblers may learn to increase the duration of this experience thereby adding to the pleasure obtained.

To return to the question of whether such periods of "unconscious" gambling represent genuine impaired control, the tracking data and direct observation accounts of regular EGM players (Haw, 2000; Walker, 2004) confirms that sessions of an hour and more comprise periods of continuous play interspersed with breaks when the player visits the bar, changes machines, goes to the toilet, smokes a cigarette (in most Australian jurisdictions requiring movement to a separate smoking environment). The autonomous player may be engrossed in play, lose track of time, stop gaming when self-awareness returns, join friends for a drink, go elsewhere, all without concerns about their gambling behaviour. Where there is impairment of self-control, is the key difference the greater salience of the emotional experience during gambling in contrast to most or all other current sources of positive emotion, and is the behaviour prioritised by innate cortical structures and functions?

As regular gambling becomes established as a regular recreational activity, is the primary theme, as suggested by Davies (1992), that gambling becomes a very pleasurable activity and is therefore sought out by the individual? When, for whatever reasons, efforts are made to limit or stop gambling, the choice is one of conflict, of approach-avoidance where the attraction is greatest within the venue stimulus complex (well illustrated by Orford (2001, p. 262)): venues that may be visited "just for a drink, to watch the game on the big screen; I won't play the pokies tonight." The likelihood of choosing to gamble varies, increasing if the prevailing mood is frustration or dysphoria and subsequent to imbibing two or more standard drinks of alcohol (Baron & Dickerson, 1999). Certainly, many regular gamblers (over a third) report difficulty in refraining from starting to gamble once near a venue (O'Connor & Dickerson, 2003).

Approach to the venue and the start of a session of gaming will be open to the influence of the cognitive processes implicated in the literature of problem gambling (Wagenaar, 1988; Griffiths, 1990; Ladouceur & Walker, 1996). Do these beliefs in skill, in winning, serve essentially to disguise the fact, to render more palatable, the fact that the player is choosing not to exert control (Edwards & Gross, 1976)? Once started, during the session itself a similar pattern may recur between periods of focused play. The player may decide to stop gambling, buy a drink at the bar and then find that the attraction of the certain strong, pleasurable, emotions contingent on returning to play are "irresistible". This attraction may alter during a lengthy session, may perhaps habituate, only to be replaced by the certain expectation of the strong negative emotions that will be experienced on stopping the session of gambling, including powerful regret if finishing behind, or before a machine is "due" to payout or a favoured horse is scheduled to run (O'Connor & Dickerson, 1997).

Some problem gamblers report "finding myself at a machine, in the venue" with no awareness of a conscious decision or struggle to make their preferred choice. Repeated internal debates leading to "failures" to exert control may become aversive (Maddern, 2004) and avoidance an understandable but unproductive coping strategy.

E. My gambling is very difficult to control even though it causes several problems.
F. My gambling is impossible to control and it causes several, significant problems that are distressing.

It is likely that the perceived enjoyment, the expected positive emotion from gambling is at its peak at the time when the negative impacts of gambling have begun to occur (Ben-Tovim et al., 2001). Once a phase has begun where the regular gambling contributes to the increased likelihood of dysphoric mood and undermines alternative sources of positive emotion (e.g. the disruption of family and marital relationships), then further impairment of self-control seems inevitable. The extreme impaired self-control items (E and F) endorsed during an assessment away from the venue, suggest that there is indeed a point at which gamblers, despite an awareness of the consequences, despite their best efforts, find it extremely difficult to impose self-restraint over their gambling.

One counter argument is that the experience of impaired control is not more than a convenient attribution or excuse. Davies (1992), for example, argued that " *'addiction' is not so much a thing that happens to people, as a functional set of cognitions surrounding the activity of taking drugs; a way of thinking made necessary only by the sanctions with which we surround the act of taking substances to change our state of consciousness*" (p. 167). In the absence of a psychoactive agent, particularly in a community and social context generally accepting gambling, such arguments are not persuasive accounts of the reports of impaired self-control of gamblers. To the outside observer, the movement of the player between machines, to the bar, may nonetheless appear opportunities for choice. In reality, the experience at these moments may be very similar to the person wanting to leave a live-in relationship. Cool, rational appraisal of the overall harmful nature of the relationship, its disruption of other friendships, its abusive aspects, may lead to the packing of bags. Yet how many have stood in hallways only to turn and fix a coffee or pour a drink and stay? How many have never tried leaving knowing that they cannot? In the context of psychological literature on addictive behaviour "to lack the strength", "to be weak", sounds pejorative; in common parlance it sounds genuine and human.

To glibly offer an explanation that emotive-laden behaviours all boil down to simply making a choice at any given time (a cognitive-reductionist approach), ignores the wealth of research and theorising that points to humans as not economically driven and rational in their decision-making, but rather as frequently messy and muddled, inconsistent and vacillating (Orford, 2001). The notion of impaired control does not of course eliminate decision-making, but calls for a continuum approach to the quality of decisions, so that at the time of giving in to an intense desire to gamble (or to sate other appetites), emotive decisions can be construed as "degraded" decisions that lack clarity and quality reasoning. As one punter put it (and readily endorsed by others in a focus group), "I continue to bet against my better judgement" (O'Connor et al., 1995).

Implications for Pathological Gambling

The results from the measurement of impaired self-control reported in Chapter 2 pose significant problems for the Pathways Model of problem gambling (Blaszczynski & Nower, 2002). The evidence from a mathematical psychology approach that impaired self-control of gambling is a quantifiable dimension from no impairment to "my gambling is impossible to control ..." (Kyngdon, 2004) was derived from participants representing the whole range of gambling involvement, infrequent players, regular gamblers *and* a clinical group of diagnosed pathological gamblers. Using the same group data from a traditional psychometric approach (SGC, 12-item version) was shown to reveal similar item response curves for all three groups of respondents.

This evidence suggests that impaired self-control of gambling is a continuous quantitative dimension ranging from autonomous no impairment to impaired control despite significant effort. The impairment experienced at lower levels differs in degree or frequency from higher levels of impairment. There was no support for a qualitatively different type of impaired self-control being reported/experienced by the clinical group of pathological gamblers.

Blaszczynski & Nower (2002) specified that "real" impaired control occurs in the context of:

1. Repeated unsuccessful attempts to resist the urge.
2. A genuine desire to cease to gamble.
3. Emergence of negative consequences.

In contrast, the evidence is that the dimension of impaired self-control is typified by increasing frequency and intensity of behavioural excess and urges to gamble respectively. Even at relatively low levels of impairment gamblers may "feel a need to control my gambling" (items B and C; Kyngdon, 2004). In fact the work on temptation–restraint both for gambling and other addictive behaviours (e.g. Collins, 1997) and the qualitative work supporting the "limit maintenance model" (Maddern, 2004) suggest that identifying a need for limits is one of the very first steps in the process of erosion of self-control. As impairment increases the inability to cut back or stop gambling for a day or a week becomes more frequent and the negative consequences increase in number and severity. The picture that emerges is that from infrequent to regular to problem gamblers, impaired self-control increases across a dimension: there is no point at which "real" impaired control appears. If this empirical picture is accurate then the distinction between Pathway I, behaviourally conditioned problem gambler, and Pathways II and III, the pathological gambler, collapses.

Aspects of the distinctive nature of behaviourally conditioned gamblers (Pathway I) specified by Blaszczynski & Nower (2002) derive from assumptions that do not match the data base presented in this monograph mainly because of their failure to distinguish regular from infrequent gamblers. For example: *"Learning theories ... fail to explain why only a small proportion of the total population of gamblers lose control."* (p. 487)

In fact amongst *regular* gamblers, where one would expect the effects of conditioning to be the strongest, impaired self-control as measured by the SGC is almost normally distributed: e.g. 43% "sometimes", "often" or "always" "feel an irresistible urge to continue gambling". Once this empirical finding is known, the high proportion of regular gamblers using continuous forms that are at risk of experiencing significant negative consequences arising from their gambling (about one in five; Productivity Commission, 1999) comes as no surprise. In contrast, Blaszczynski & Nower (2002) assume that impaired control *is rare* and therefore have to find other reasons for the occurrence of negative consequences amongst regular gamblers. They propose that the harm arises from bad judgement and poor decision-making. Such cognitive processes may contribute to negative consequences amongst gamblers at all levels of involvement, but where impaired self-control is common and a strong correlate of harm, why would one expect bad judgement and poor decision-making to always operate as a strong causal factor (as opposed to equally, or more often, being a consequence of losing control)? As we have suggested with reference to other cognitive variables, such poor decision-making needs more careful definition and measurement to permit empirical evidence to be gathered.

Another assumption of the Pathways Model is that for the behaviourally conditioned gambler (Pathway I) the negative impacts arising from the gambling are *"consequences not the cause of excessive gambling"* (p. 487). Such a distinction is impossible to sustain particularly in the context of the role of negative mood on impaired control: such non-clinical levels of mood could arise from a variety of sources such as vocational, relationship and financial concerns and it would be impossible to determine whether the gambling had been a contributing factor or not. In the "first instance" in youth gamblers the failure, repeatedly, to stick to limits of time and money expenditure does result in a complex of negative emotions, guilt and self-blame, but this rapidly seems to become an expectation of failure and further impaired control (Maddern, 2004).

In summary, the research described in this monograph has provided a more detailed picture of Pathway I, the behaviourally conditioned gambler, and in so doing has undermined Blaszczynski & Nower's (2002) definition of pathological gamblers who experience "real" impaired control. The model reduces to a single pathway, the behaviourally conditioned gambler, plus two categories of risk factors that increase either or both the level of impaired self-control and the probability that the negative impacts of gambling will be numerous and severe.

What is no longer clear is quite where pathological gambling begins. If the authors wish to retain the concept of pathological gambling arising from distinctive and separate pathways from regular gamblers they will need to provide evidence of "real" impaired control or to define alternative distinguishing characteristics. Their framework remains a valuable integration of existing knowledge about problem gambling, a framework for future research that still avoids being *"a misguided venture ... of ... applying one theoretical model to pathological gambling"* (Blaszczynski & Nower, 2002, p. 487), but the model will profit from greater emphasis on a continuum approach to impaired control and an acknowledgement that such impairment is a *common* experience of regular gamblers.

Implications for Problem Gambling Policy

It was concluded that the current policy of "responsible gambling" (e.g. the "Reno Model", Blaszczynski et al., 2004) inappropriately places the emphasis on the individual regular gambler to learn to not gamble excessively, to maintain self-control. Even in the absence of data on impaired control the speed, complexity and potentially unending sequence of opportunities to purchase the gambling product (e.g. EGMs, off-course betting and casino table games) suggests a failure to comply with established principles of consumer protection.

In this context the data on impaired self-control presented in this monograph merely confirms what would be expected of individuals who spend several hours a week purchasing such gambling products and provides the underlying explanation of why such gamblers have been assessed to be the most "at risk" of all consumers of gambling (Productivity Commission, 1999).

It is inappropriate for harm prevention policy to expect that such gamblers, whose losses may account for up to 85% of all gambling expenditure, maintain control simply by providing them with information: the data on impaired control was in fact gathered in a jurisdiction where such education has been available for some years in the media and in the venues and even pasted to the EGMs, to the note acceptor. In the same way that now we can look back on the "dark" days before compulsory wearing of seatbelts and random breath testing, when the responsibility for safety was by means of driver education, so too may the next generation of gambling experts, the industry, the community and governments look back in judgement on the contemporary failure to provide gamblers with the technological means to stick to their chosen budgets, preferring instead to promote the myth of "responsible gambling".

Implications for Addiction

The issue addressed in this final section is whether the body of work completed on impaired self-control of gambling has any implications for research and theory of addictive behaviours generally. In other words have the emerging results gone any way toward answering the challenge of Orford? *"If thinking about addiction is going to change, the study of excessive gambling is likely to be one of the richest sources of new ideas."* (Orford, 2001, p. 3)

The apparently "artificial" separation of impaired self-control of gambling from its resultant harmful impacts has shown some promise. The conceptualisation and definition of impaired self-control, whether in the context of unfolding theory and mathematical psychology, or traditional psychometric measurement has confirmed that it is a significant quantifiable dimension meriting study in its own right. Although items describing impaired self-control of gambling readily combine with other addictive cognitive and behavioural themes paralleling established models in other addictive behaviours (e.g. Collins, 1997; Maddern, 2004), in so doing the psychological processes underlying the erosion of self-control may be obscured.

This is not to conclude that models such as the temptation–restraint are not valuable: they are important conceptualisations that aid our understanding and generate important implications for treatment and prevention. The point is that impaired self-control as the key factor in a psychological conceptualisation of addictive behaviours demands theoretical and research evaluation as a unique dimension. This is not an original suggestion, as much of the foundation for the present work on gambling was derived from similar arguments made by Heather et al. (1993) for problem drinking. The conclusions we have drawn regarding problem gambling reinforce the argument that perhaps concepts such as the Alcohol Dependence Syndrome, in which impaired control was only one of seven elements, most of which related to proposed biochemical neuroadaptive processes, may have arisen from an overly medical concept of dependence and/or over-reliance on the methods of factor analysis (Kyngdon & Dickerson, 2005), thereby resulting in models that obscure the potentially unique addictive themes associated with impaired control.

In the absence of the complexity of a psychoactive agent, an essentially normal learning account of problem gambling was shown to be a potentially powerful explanation of impaired control and the range of resulting negative consequences. Hours and frequency of practice reinforced by salient emotions erode self-control, which is exacerbated by prior dysphoric mood particularly in women, and alcohol intake and individual differences in impulsivity in men.

Speculative parallels with other addictive behaviours can readily be drawn. The emphasis on salient emotion as the reinforcement may be supported by the evidence from the Stroop test: the effect has been shown for other addictive behaviours (e.g. Green et al., 1999; Stormark et al., 2000) and for "pathological gambling" and impaired control of gambling behaviour amongst regular EGM players (McCusker & Gettings, 1997; Boyer & Dickerson, 2003, respectively). The emphasis on emotion is perhaps the most important theme for the addictive behaviours to emerge from the current work on gambling. If conditioning involving salient emotion is suggested to be the start of the erosion of self-control, then links are immediately apparent with two essentially psychological accounts of the addictions:

I. In "classic texts revisited" Heather (2004) drew attention to the potential theoretical importance for the addictions of the work of Ainslie (1975) who argued that impulsivity, that is, in the present context "impaired self-control", was a function of an innate preference for the small-early reward over the large-later rather than acquired from the organism's conditioning history. The data from gambling suggests that *both* mechanisms may be involved. The conditioning of the behavioural emotion outcome strengthens the attraction of the small-early reward, and the fact that the reward is emotional provides the link with potential innate mechanisms that have primacy over decision-making cognitive processes, for example the emotion control precedence of Frijda (1986) whereby emotion can "*override other concerns, other goals and actions* ... (and) *considerations of appropriateness of long-term consequences*" (p. 355). Thus, the emphasis on emotion supports the key theme presented by Ainslie, that the addictive "struggle" is the attempt to forestall the naturally prioritised impulsive actions that the individual knows will occur under certain conditions.

II. Orford's (2001) psychological view of the addictions is a far more comprehensive psychological account and is centred on the concept of attachment to appetitive behaviour to a level of excess. Strong attachment arises from the association of the behaviour with strong emotions, both positive and negative. Eventually the behaviour comes to provide access not just to arousal and pleasure, but also an escape from anger and depression arising from the consequences of the behaviour. In the current work on gambling, the focus on impaired self-control limited the examination of the "feedback" effects of the consequences of the excessive gambling on further impaired control.

A critical difference between gambling and other addictive behaviours is that the former, at least for the types of gambling known to be the most difficult to control, the continuous forms, all occur in special environments with set temporal patterns of stimuli leading up to the gambling response, the button press, bet placement. One might speculate that where there is a psychoactive agent the addictive response such as taking a drink, drawing on a cigarette, injecting a vein, may be set in a somewhat variable sequence of stimuli that can occur in a variety of environments. If conditioning is also a key process for such addictive behaviours then the repetition of an exact sequence of cues may be less a requirement of strong conditioning simply because the effective timing of the reinforcing salient positive emotional experience is consistently triggered by the process of ingestion per se. In gambling, given the emotional response is itself acquired by being paired with the possibility of winning money, the preceding sequence of stimuli are entirely fixed. Either the gambling response can only occur just before the onset of the emotional experience (e.g. as with EGMs) or, as we have speculated in the off-course betting venue sequence, gambling responses are shaped to occur as late as possible in the cycle by the greater efficacy of reinforcement for such late staking.

The extraordinarily contrived and regulated nature of much contemporary gambling, where by design there is repetition of temporal sequences of stimuli that give pleasure whilst eroding self-control, provides an explanation why few other behaviours, not involving a psychoactive drug or substance (e.g. food), become so strongly, and rapidly, addictive.

In this monograph the emphasis has been on the natural, non-pathological psychological processes. In such a conceptual framework the addictive behaviours risk losing some of their unique character. Is it satisfactory or adequate to view such excessive behaviours as the outcome of very effective emotional conditioning? The behaviours themselves are all relatively simple and readily acquired, but after conditioning consistently provide access to salient positive emotion. Where else in human endeavours, in relationships, in parenting, in work, in play, are such simple dependable responses available to access similar salient positive emotion? Strong positive emotions tend to emerge in any such domain from a complex of responses over long periods of time, the hard yards of common duties, often unpredictably, such as the glimpse of one's child at play, the glance of a lover, the well-struck winner, the spontaneous approval of workmates. These large-later rewards may bring joy, but when competing with the small-early rewards of the addictions they require "precommitment" strategies (Ainslie, 1975), such as relationship vows, parental promises and social sanctions to prevent innate impulsive choices. Sirens may be less common, but like Odysseus, we are still having ourselves tied to a mast as temptations become ever more accessible.

References

Aasved, M. (2003). *The Biology of Gambling*. Springfield, Illinois: Charles C. Thomas.

Abbott, M.W. & Volberg, R.A. (1992). *Frequent gamblers and problem gamblers in New Zealand*. Research Series No. 14. Wellington: Department of Internal Affairs.

Abbott, M.W., Williams, M.M. & Volberg, R.A. (1999). *Seven years on: a follow-up study of frequent and problem gamblers living in the community*. Report No. 2 of the New Zealand Gaming Survey. Wellington, New Zealand: Department of Internal Affairs.

ACIL (2001). *The impact of gaming in Ballarat*, commissioned by Tattersall's, cited in Banks (2003).

Ainslie, G. (1975). Specious reward: a behavioural theory of impulsiveness and impulse control. *Psychological Bulletin*, 82, 463–496.

Allcock, C. (Ed.) (2002). *Current Issues Related to Identifying the Problem Gambler in the Gambling Venue*. Melbourne: Australian Gaming Council (AGC).

Allcock, C. & Dickerson, M.G. (1986). *The Guide to Good Gambling*. Wentworth Falls, NSW: Social Sciences Press.

American Gaming Association (AGA) (1998). *Responsible Gaming Resource Guide* (2nd edn.). Washington DC: American Gaming Association.

American Psychiatric Association (APA) (1980). *Diagnostic and Statistical Manual of Mental Disorders* (3rd edn.). Washington DC: American Psychiatric Association.

American Psychiatric Association (APA) (1994). *Diagnostic and Statistical Manual of Mental Disorders* (4th edn.). Washington DC: American Psychiatric Association.

Anderson, G. & Brown, R.I.F. (1984). Real and laboratory gambling: sensation-seeking and arousal. *British Journal of Psychology*, 75, 401–410.

Australian Bureau of Statistics (ABS) (1997). *Australia Now – a Statistical Profile*. Canberra: Commonwealth of Australia.

Australian Bureau of Statistics (ABS) (2003). *Population by Age and Sex*. Cat. 3201.0, Canberra: Australian Bureau of Statistics.

Azmier, J. (2001). *Gambling in Canada 2001: An Overview*. Calgary, AB: Canada West Foundation.

Babor, T.F., de la Fuente, J.R., Saunders, J. & Grant, M. (1992). Programme on substance abuse. *AUDIT the Alcohol Disorders Identification Test: Guidelines for Use in Primary Health Care.* World Health Organisation Publication No. 92.4. Geneva: World Health Organisation.

Banks, G. (2003). The productivity commission's gambling inquiry: 3 years on, gambling research. (*Journal of the National Association for Gambling Studies, Australia*), 15, 7–28.

Barbeyrac, J. (1737). Traite du Jeu (3 vols), Amsterdam (cited by Oxford, 2001).

Barnes, G.M., Welte, J.W., Hoffman, J.H. & Dintcheff, B.A. (1999). Gambling and alcohol use among youth: influences of demographic, socialization, and individual factors. *Addictive Behaviors*, 24(6), 749–767.

Baron, J. (1994). *Thinking and Deciding.* Cambridge: Cambridge University Press.

Baron, E. & Dickerson, M.D. (1999). Alcohol consumption and self-control of gambling behaviour. *Journal of Gambling Studies*, 15, 3–15.

Baron, R.M. & Kenny, D.A. (1986). The moderator – mediator variable distinction in social psychological research: conceptual, strategic and statistical considerations. *Journal of Personality and Social Psychology*, 51(6), 1173–1182.

Baron, E., Dickerson, M.D. & Blaszczynski, A. (1995). The scale of gambling choices: preliminary development of an instrument to measure impaired control of gambling behaviour. In O'Connor, J. (Ed.), *High Stakes in the Nineties*. National Association of Gambling Studies, Curtin University Press (pp. 153–167).

Barrera, M., Sandler, I.N. & Ramsay, T.B. (1981). Preliminary development of a scale of social support: studies on college students. *American Journal of Community Psychology*, 9(4), 435–447.

Battersby, M. & Tolchard, B. (1996). The effect of treatment on pathological gamblers referred to a behavioural psychotherapist unit: I – Changes in psychiatric co-morbidity after treatment. In Tolchard, B. (Ed.), *Towards 2000: The Future of Gambling*. Proceedings of the 7th Conference of the National Association for Gambling Studies, Adelaide. Melbourne: National Association for Gambling Studies (pp. 53–57).

Baumeister, R.F. (1997). Esteem threat, self-regulatory breakdown, and emotional distress as factors in self-defeating behaviour. *Review of General Psychology*, 1(2), 145–174.

Beaudoin, C.M. & Cox, C.J. (1999). Characteristics of problem gambling in a Canadian context: a preliminary study using a DSM-IV-based questionnaire. *Canadian Journal of Psychiatry*, 44, 483–487.

Ben-Tovim, D.I., Esterman, A., Tolchard, B. & Battersby, M. (2001). *The Victorian Gambling Screen*. Melbourne, Vic.: Gambling Research Panel (ISBN 07 311 1440X).

Bergh, C. & Kulhorn, C. (1994). Social, psychological and physical consequences of pathological gambling in Sweden. *Journal of Gambling Studies*, 10(3), 275–285.

Bergh, C., Ekland, T., Sodersten, P. & Nordin, C. (1997). Altered dopamine function in pathological gambling. *Psychological Medicine*, 27, 473–475.

Bergler, E. (1957). *The Psychology of Gambling*. New York: Hill & Wang.

Black, R. & Ramsay, H. (2003). The ethics of gambling: guidelines for players and commercial providers. *International Gambling Studies*, 3(2), 199–216.

Blaszczynski, A. (1998). *Overcoming Compulsive Gambling; a Self-help Guide Using Cognitive Behavioural Techniques.* London: Robinson Publishing.

Blaszczynski, A. & McConaghy, N. (1988). *Pathological Gambling and Criminal Behaviour.* Report to Criminology Research Council, Canberra.

Blaszczynski, A. & Nower, L. (2002). A pathways model of problem and pathological gambling. *Addiction,* 97(5), 487–499.

Blaszczynski, A., Buhrich, N. & McConaghy, N. (1985). Pathological gamblers, heroin addicts and controls compared on the E.P.Q. "Addiction Scale". *British Journal of Addiction,* 80, 315–319.

Blaszczynski, A., McConaghy, N. & Frankova, A. (1991a). Control versus abstinence in the treatment of pathological gambling: a two to nine year follow-up. *British Journal of Addiction,* 86(3), 299–306.

Blaszczynski, A., McConaghy, N. & Frankova, A. (1991b). A comparison of relapsed and non-relapsed abstinent pathological gamblers following behavioural treatment. *British Journal of Addiction,* 86, 1485–1489.

Blaszczynski, A., Steel, Z. & McConaghy, N. (1997) Impulsivity in pathological gambling: the antisocial impulsivist. Addiction, 92, 75–87.

Blaszczynski, A., Sharpe, L. & Walker, M. (2001). *The assessment of the impact of the reconfiguration on electronic gaming machines as harm minimisation strategies for problem gambling.* A Report for the Gaming Industry Operators Group. Sydney: UOS Printing Service.

Blaszczynski, A., Ladouceur, R. & Shaffer, H. (2004). A science based framework for responsible gambling: the Reno model. *Journal of Gambling Studies,* 20(3), 301–317.

Bohn, M.J., Babor, T.F. & Kranzler, H.R. (1995). The alcohol use disorders identification test (AUDIT): validation of a screening instrument for use in medical settings. *Journal of Studies on Alcohol,* 56(4), 423–432.

Boyer, M. & Dickerson, M.G. (2003). Attentional bias and addictive behaviour: automaticity in a gambling specific modified Stroop task. *Addiction,* 98, 61–70.

Breen, R.B. & Zimmerman, M. (2002). Rapid onset of pathological gambling in machine gamblers. *Journal of Gambling Studies,* 18, 31–43.

Breen, B. & Zuckerman, M. (1999). Chasing in gambling behaviour: personality and cognitive determinants. *Personality and Individual Differences,* 27, 1097–1111.

Breiter, H.C., Aharon, I., Kahneman, D., Dale, A. & Shizgal, P. (2001). Functional imaging of neural responses to expectancy and experience of monetary gains and losses. *Neuron,* 30, 619–639.

Brockner, J. & Rubin, J.Z. (1985). *Entrapment in escalating conflicts: a social psychological analysis.* New York: Springer-Verlag.

Brown, L. (1993). *The New Shorter Oxford Dictionary.* Oxford: Clarendon Press.

Brown, R.I.F. (1986). Arousal and sensation seeking components in the general explanation of gambling and gambling addictions. *International Journal of Addictions,* 21(9 & 10), 1001–1016.

Brown, R.I.F. (1987). Gambling addictions, arousal and an affective/decision-making explanation of behavioural reversions or relapses. *International Journal of Addictions*, 22(11), 1053–1067.

Browne, B.R. (1989). Going on tilt: frequent poker players and control. *Journal of Gambling Studies*, 5(1), 3–21.

Bryson, W. (2004). *A Short History of Nearly Everything*. London: Blackswan.

Carver, C.S., Scheier, M.F. & Weintraub, J.K. (1989). Assessing coping strategies: a theoretically based approach. *Journal of Personality and Social Psychology*, 56 (2), 267–283.

Catania, A.C. (1998). *Learning* (4th edn.). New Jersey: Prentice-Hall.

Chance, P. (1994). *Learning and Behaviour* (3rd edn.). California: Brooks Cole.

Charlton, P. (1987). *Two Flies Up a Wall: The Australian Passion for Gambling*. Sydney: Methuen Haynes.

Chesher, G. & Greeley, J. (1989). The effect of alcohol on cognitive and psychomotor functioning. In Greeley, J. & Gladstone, W. (Eds), *National Drug and Alcohol Research Centre Monograph No 8*. Sydney: National Drug and Alcohol Research Centre (pp. 47–98).

Ciarrocchi, J. (1987). Severity of impairment in dually addicted gamblers. *Journal of Gambling Behavior*, 3(1), 16–26.

Ciarrocchi, J. & Richardson, R. (1989). Profile of compulsive gamblers in treatment: update and comparisons. *Journal of Gambling Behavior*, 5(1), 53–65.

Cocco, N., Sharpe, L. & Blaszczynski, A. (1995). Differences in the preferred level of arousal in two sub-groups of problem gamblers: a preliminary report. *Journal of Gambling Studies*, 11(2), 221–229.

Collins, R.L. (1997). Drinking restraint and risk for alcohol abuse. In Marlatt, G.A. & Vandenbos, G.R. (Eds), *Addictive Behaviors: Readings on Etiology, Prevention and Treatment*. Washington DC: American Psychiatric Association (pp. 289–306).

Collins, R.L. & Lapp, W.M. (1992). The temptation and restraint inventory for measuring drinking restraint. *British Journal of Addiction*, 87(4), 625–633.

Collins, R.L., Lapp, W.M. & Izzo, C.V. (1994). Affective and behavioural reactions to violation of limits on alcohol consumption. *Journal of Studies on Alcohol*, 55(4) 475–486.

Collins, W.A., Laursen, B., Mortensen, N., Luebbker, C. & Ferriera, M. (1997). Conflict processes and transitions in parent and peer relationships: implications for autonomy and regulation. *Journal of Adolescent Research*, 12(2), 178–198.

Comings, D.E., Rosenthal, R., Lesieur, H.R., Rugle, L.J., Muhleman, D., Chiu, C., Dietz, G. & Gade, R. (1996). A study of the dopamine D2 receptor gene in pathological gambling. *Pharmacogenetics*, 6(3), 223–234.

Connors, G.J., Collins, R.L., Dermen, K.H. & Koutsky, J.R. (1998). Substance use restraint: an extension of the construct to a clinical population. *Cognitive Therapy and Research*, 22(1), 75–87.

Coombs, C.H. (1950). Psychological scaling without a unit of measurement. *Psychological Review*, 57, 145–158.

Coombs, C.H. (1964). *A Theory of Data*. New York: Wiley.

Coombs, C.H. (1975). A note on the relation between the vector model and the unfolding model for preferences. *Psychometrica*, 40, 115–116.

Coombs, C.H. & Kao, R.C. (1960). On a connection between factor analysis and multidimensional unfolding. *Psychometrica*, 25, 219–231.

Corless, T. & Dickerson, M.G. (1989). Gamblers' self-perceptions and the determinants of impaired control. *British Journal of Addiction*, 84, 1527–1537.

Corney, W.J. & Cummings, W.T. (1985). Gambling behaviour and information processing biases. *Journal of Gambling Behavior*, 1(2) 111–118.

Cornish, D.B. (1978). *Gambling: A Review of the Literature and its Implications for Policy and Research*. London: HMSO.

Costa, P.T. & McCrae, R.R. (1992a). *The Revised NEO Personality Inventory (NEO-PI-R) and NEO Five-Factor Inventory (NEO-FFI) Professional Manual*. Odessa, Florida: Psychological Assessment Resources.

Costa, P.T. & McCrae, R.R. (1992b). Trait psychology comes of age. In Sonderegger, T.B. (Ed.), *Nebraska Symposium on Motivation: Psychology and Ageing*. Lincoln, New England: University of Nebraska Press.

Costello, T. & Millar, R. (2000). *Wanna Bet? Winners and Losers in Gambling's Luck Myth*. Sydney: Allen & Unwin.

Coventry, K.R. & Brown, R.I.F. (1993). Sensation seeking, gambling and gambling addictions. *Addiction*, 88, 541–554.

Coventry, K. & Hudson, J. (2001). Gender differences, physiological arousal and the role of winning in fruit machine gamblers. *Addiction*, 96(6), 871–879.

Coventry, K.R. & Norman, A.C. (1997). Arousal, sensation seeking and frequency of gambling in off-course racing bettors. *British Journal of Psychology*, 88, 671–681.

Culleton, R.P. (1989). The prevalence rates of pathological gambling: a look at methods. *Journal of Gambling Behavior*, 5(1), 22–41.

Cunningham-Williams, R.M., Cottler, L.B., Compton, W.M. & Spitznagel, E.L. (1998). Taking chances: problem gamblers and mental health disorders – results from the St. Louis Epidemiologic Catchment Area study. *American Journal of Public Health*, 88(7), 1093–1096.

Custer, R.L. (1982). Pathological Gambling. In Whitfield, A. (Ed.), *Patients with Alcoholism and Other Drug Problems*. New York: Year Book Publishers (pp.76–102).

Custer, R.L. (1984). Profile of the pathological gambler. *Journal of Clinical Psychiatry*, 45, 35–38.

Daghestani, A.N., Elenz, E. & Crayton, J.W. (1996). Pathological gambling in hospitalized substance abusing veterans. *Journal of Clinical Psychiatry*, 57(8), 360–363.

Davey, G. (1989). *Ecological Learning Theory*. Great Britain: Routledge.

Davies, D.L. (1962). Normal drinking in recovered alcoholics. *Quarterly Journal of Alcohol Studies*, 23, 94–104.

Davies, J.B. (1992). *The myth of addiction*. Chur, Switzerland: Harwood.

Deci, E.L. & Ryan, R.N. (1985). The support of autonomy and the control of behavior. *Journal of Personality and Social Psychology*, 53, 1024–1027.

De Fuentes-Merrillas, L., Koeler, L.W.J., Bethlehem, J., Schipers, G.M. & VanDenBrink, W. (2003). Are scratch cards addictive? The prevalence of scratch card addiction in the Netherlands. *Addiction*, 98(6), 725–732.

Delfabbro, P.H. & Winefield, A.H. (1999). Poker-machine gambling: an analysis of within session characteristics. *British Journal of Psychology*, 90, 425–439.

Delfabbro, P.H. & Winefield, A.H. (2000). Predictors of irrational thinking in regular slot machine gamblers. *The Journal of Psychology*, 134, 117–128.

Department of Human Services (DHS) (1999). *The impacts of gambling on adolescents and children*. Melbourne: Department of Human Services.

Department of Human Services (DHS) (2000). *Playing for time: exploring the impacts of gambling on women*. Melbourne: Department of Human Services.

Department of Internal Affairs (2001). *What do we know about gambling and problem gambling in New Zealand?* Report No. 7 of the New Zealand Gaming Survey. Wellington: Department of Internal Affairs.

Derevensky, J.L., Gupta, R. & Cioppa, J.D. (1996). A developmental perspective of gambling behavior in children and adolescents. *Journal of Gambling Behavior*, 12(1), 49–56.

Dickerson, M.G. (1979). FI schedules and persistence at gambling in the UK betting office. *Journal of Applied Behavior Analysis*, 12, 315–323.

Dickerson, M.G. (1991). Internal and external determinants of persistent gambling. In Heather, N., Miller, W.M. & Greeley, J. (Eds), *Self Control and the Addictive Behaviours*. Sydney: Maxwell McMillan. (pp. 317–338).

Dickerson, M.G. (1993). A preliminary exploration of a 2-stage method in the assessment of the extent and degree of gambling related problems in the Australian community. In Eadington, W., Cornelius, J. & Taber, J. (Eds), *Gambling Behaviour and Problem Gambling*. Reno Institute for the Study of Gambling and Commercial Gaming, University of Nevada (pp. 336–47).

Dickerson, M.G. (1999). Responsible gambling and EGM players. In Coman, G. (Ed.), *Practitioners' Conference, Adelaide*. Victoria: National Association for Gambling Studies (pp. 124–141).

Dickerson, M.G. (2003). The evolving contribution of gambling research to addiction theory (editorial). *Addiction*, 98(6), 709.

Dickerson, M.G. (2003a). *Client and service analysis*. Report No. 8. Melbourne: Department of Human Services.

Dickerson, M.G. (2003b). Exploring the limits of "responsible gambling": harm minimisation or consumer protection? *Gambling Research (Journal of the National Association for Gambling Studies, Australia)*, 15, 29–44.

Dickerson, M.G. & Adcock, S.G. (1987). Mood arousal and cognitions in persistent gambling: preliminary investigation of a theoretical model. *Journal of Gambling Behavior*, 3(1), 3–15.

Dickerson, M.G. & Baron, E. (1994a). *A baseline study of the extent and impact of gambling in Tasmania with particular reference to problem gambling by the Australian Institute for Gambling Research.* Report to Department of Treasury, Tasmanian Government. Hobart: Tasmanian Government Printer.

Dickerson, M.G. & Baron, E. (1994b). *An assessment of the extent and degree of gambling related problems in the population of Western Australian the Australian Institute for Gambling Research.* Report to the Problem Gambling Steering Committee, Western Australian Government.

Dickerson, M. & Baron, E. (2000). Contemporary issues and future directions for research into pathological gambling. *Addiction*, 95(8), 1145–1159.

Dickerson, M.G. & Weekes, D. (1979). Controlled gambling as a therapeutic technique for compulsive gamblers. *Journal of Behaviour Therapy & Experimental Psychiatry*, 10, 139–141.

Dickerson, M.G., Hinchy, J. & Fabre, J. (1987). Chasing, arousal and sensation seeking in off-course gamblers. *British Journal of Addiction*, 82, 673–680.

Dickerson, M.G., Hinchy, J. & Legg England, S. (1990). Minimal treatments and problem gamblers: a preliminary investigation. *Journal of Gambling Studies*, 6(1), 87–103.

Dickerson, M. G., Cunningham, R., Legg England, S. & Hinchy, J. (1991). On the determinants of persistent gambling III. Personality, prior mood, and poker machine play. *The International Journal of the Addictions*, 26(5), 531–548.

Dickerson, M.G., Hinchy, J., Legg England, S., Fabre, J. & Cunningham, R. (1992). On the determinants of persistent gambling I. high frequency poker machine players. *British Journal of Psychology*, 83, 237–248.

Dickerson, M.G., Allcock, C., Blaszczynski, A., Nicholls, B., Williams, J. & Maddern, R. (1996a) *Study 2: An examination of the socio-economic effects of gambling on individuals, families and the community, including research into the costs of problem gambling in New South Wales.* Report to the Casino Community Benefit Fund Trustees, NSW Government.

Dickerson, M.G., Baron, E., Hong, S.M. & Cottrell, D. (1996b). Estimating the extent and degree of gambling related problems in the Australian population: a national prevalence study. *Journal of Gambling Studies*, 12, 161–178.

Dickerson, M.G., McMillen, J., Hallebone, E., Volberg, R. & Wooley, R. (1997). *Definition and incidence of problem gambling including the socio-economic distribution.* Report to the Victorian Casino and Gaming Authority (VCGA), Victoria.

Dickerson, M.G., Allcock, C., Blaszczynski, A., Nicholls, B., Williams, J. & Maddern, R. (1998) *Study 2 (repeat): an examination of the socio-economic effects of gambling on individuals, families and the community, including research into the costs of problem gambling in New South Wales,* Report to the Casino Community Benefit Fund Trustees, NSW Government.

Dickerson, M.G., Hills, S., Wodak, A. & Mattick R. (2001). *The co-morbidity of alcohol and gambling problems in NSW.* Report to the Casino Community Benefit Fund, Department of Gaming and Racing, NSW Government, Sydney.

Di Dio, K. & Ong, B. (1997). The conceptual link between avoidant coping style, stress and problem gambling. In Coman, G., Evans, B. & Wootton, R. (Eds), *Responsible Gambling – a Future Winner.* Proceedings of the 8th. National Association for Gambling Studies Conference, Melbourne. Melbourne: the National Association for Gambling Studies (Australia) (pp. 91–100).

Diener, E. (1999). Introduction to the special section on the structure of emotion. *Journal of Personality and Social Psychology*, 76, 803–804.

Diskin, K.M. & Hodgins, D.C. (2003). Psychophysiological and subjective arousal during gambling in pathological and non-pathological video lottery gamblers. *International Gambling Studies*, 3(1), 37–51.

Diskin, K.M., Hodgins, D.C. & Skitch, S.A. (2003). Psychophysiological and subjective responses of a community sample of video lottery gamblers in gaming venues and laboratory situations. *International Gambling Studies*, 3(2), 133–148.

Dowling, N., Smith, D. & Thomas, T. (2005). Electronic gaming machines: are they the "crack-cocaine" of gambling? *Addiction*, 100, 1, 33–45.

Eadington, W. (1996). Ethical and policy considerations in the spread of commercial gambling. In McMillen, J. (Ed.) *Gambling Cultures*. London: Routledge, pp. 243–262.

Edwards, G. (1985). A later follow-up of a classic case series: D.L. Davies' 1962 report and its significance for the present. *Journal of Studies on Alcohol*, 46(3), 181–190.

Edwards, G. (1986). The alcohol dependence syndrome: a concept as stimulus to enquiry. *British Journal of Addiction*, 81, 171–183.

Edwards, G. & Gross, M.M. (1976). Alcohol dependence: provisional description of a clinical syndrome. *British Medical Journal*, 1, 1058–1061.

Edwards, G., Gross, M.M., Keller, M., Moser, J. & Room, R. (1977). *Alcohol Related Disabilities*. WHO Offset Publ. No. 32. Geneva: World Health Organisation.

Eisen, S.A., Lin, N., Lyons, M.J., Scherrer, J.F., Griffith, K., True, W.R., Goldberg, J. & Tsuang, M.T. (1998). Familial influences on gambling behavior: an analysis of 3359 twin pairs. *Addiction*, 93(9), 1375–1384.

Elia, C. & Jacobs, D.F. (1993). The incidence of pathological gambling among Native Americans treated for alcohol dependence. *International Journal of the Addictions*, 28(7), 659–666.

Endler, N.S. & Parker, J.D.A. (1990). *Coping Inventory for Stressful Situations (CISS): Manual.* Toronto: Multi Health Systems.

Epstein, E.E. (2001). Classification of alcohol-related problems and dependence. In Heather, N., Peters, T.J. & Stockwell, T. (Eds), *Alcohol Dependence and Problems*. Chichester: Wiley (pp. 34–47).

Ewen, C. L. (1932). *Lotteries and Sweepstakes: An Historical, Legal and Ethical Survey of their Introduction, Suppression, and Re-establishment in the British Isles.* London: Cranton.

Ferris, J. & Wynne, H. (2001). *The Canadian Problem Gambling Index*. Ottawa, Ontario: Canadian Centre on Substance Abuse.

Fisher, S. (1992). Measuring pathological gambling in children: the case of fruit machines in the UK. *Journal of Gambling Studies*, 8, 263–285.

Fisher, S. (2000). Developing the DSM-IV criteria to identify adolescent problem gambling in non-clinical populations. *Journal of Gambling Studies*, 16(2–3), 253–273.

Folkman, S., Lazarus, R.S., Dunkel-Schetter, C., DeLongis, A. & Gruen, R. (1986). Dynamics of a stressful encounter: cognitive appraisal, coping and encounter outcomes. *Journal of Personality and Social Psychology*, 50(5), 992–1003.

Frijda, N.H. (1986). *The Emotions*. Cambridge: Cambridge University Press.

Frydenberg, E. & Lewis, R. (1997). *Coping Scale for Adults, Administrators' Manual: Research Edition*. Melbourne, Australia: Australian Council for Educational Research.

Gaboury, A. & Ladouceur, R. (1989). Erroneous perceptions and gambling. *Journal of Social Behaviour and Personality*, 4, 411–420.

Gambling Research Panel (GRP) (2003a). *Best practice in problem gambling services*. GRP Report No. 3. Melbourne: Gambling Research Panel.

Gambling Research Panel (GRP) (2003b). *Evaluation of self-exclusion programme*. GRP Report No. 2. Melbourne: Gambling Research Panel.

Gambling Research Panel (GRP) (2003c). *Measuring problem gambling-evaluation of the Victorian Gambling Screen*. GRP Report No. 4. Melbourne: Gambling Research Panel.

Gambling Research Panel (GRP) (2004). *2003 Victorian longitudinal attitudes survey*. GRP Report No. 6. Melbourne: Gambling Research Panel.

Goffman, E. (1969). *Where The Action is*. London: Allen Lane.

Goldstein, H. (1995). *Multilevel Statistical Models*. London: Edward Arnold.

Green, J. & Shellingberger, R. (1991). *The Dynamics of Health and Wellness: A Biopsychosocial Approach*. Fort Worth: Holt Rinehart Winston.

Green, M., Corr, P. & De Silva, L. (1999). Impaired colour naming of body shape-related words in anorexia nervosa: affective valence or associative priming? *Cognitive Therapy and Research*, 23, 413–422.

Greenberg, J.L., Lewis, S.E. & Dodd, D.K. (1999). Overlapping addictions and self-esteem among college men and women. *Addictive Behaviors*, 24(4), 565–571.

Griffiths, M.D. (1990). The cognitive psychology of gambling. *Journal of Gambling Studies*, 6(1), 31–42.

Griffiths, M.D. (1991a). The psychobiology of the near-miss in fruit machine gambling. *Journal of Psychology*, 125, 347–357.

Griffiths, M.D. (1991b). The observational study of adolescent gambling in UK amusement arcades. *Journal of Community and Applied Social Psychology*, 1(4), 309–320.

Griffiths, M.D. (1993a). Factors in adolescent problem fruit machine gambling. *Journal of Gambling Studies*, 9, 31–45.

Griffiths, M.D. (1993b). Fruit machine gambling: the importance of structural characteristics. *Journal of Gambling Studies*, 9(2), 101–120.

Griffiths, M.D. (1994a). An exploratory study of gambling cross-addictions. *Journal of Gambling Studies*, 10(4), 371–384.

Griffiths, M.D. (1994b). The role of cognitive bias and skill in fruit machine gambling. *British Journal of Psychology*, 85, 351–369.

Griffiths, M.D. (1995a). *Adolescent Gambling*. London: Routledge.

Griffiths, M.D. (1995b). The role of subjective mood states in the maintenance of gambling behaviour. *Journal of Gambling Studies*, 11, 123–135.

Griffiths, M.D. (1996). Pathological gambling: a review of the literature. *Journal of Psychiatric and Mental Health Nursing*, 3, 347–353.

Griffiths, M.D. (1999a). Internet addiction: fact or fiction? *The Psychologist: Bulletin of the British Psychological Society*, 12, 246–250.

Griffiths, M.D. (1999b). The psychology of the near-miss revisited: a comment on DelFabbro and Winefield. *British Journal of Psychology*, 90(3), 441–445.

Grolnick, W.S. & Ryan, R.M. (1987). Autonomy in children's learning: an experimental and individual difference investigation. *Journal of Personality and Social Psychology*, 52(5), 890–898.

Gupta, R. & Derevensky, J.L. (1997). Familial and social influences on juvenile gambling behavior. *Journal of Gambling Studies*, 13(3), 179–192.

Gupta, R. & Derevensky, J.L. (1998). Adolescent gambling behaviour: a prevalence study and an examination of the correlates associated with problem gambling. *Journal of Gambling Studies*, 14(4), 319–345.

Hardoon, K.K. & Derevensky, J.L. (2002). Child and adolescent gambling behaviour: current knowledge. *Clinical Child Psychology and Psychiatry*, 7(2), 263–281.

Haw, J. (2000). *An operant analysis of gaming machine play*. Unpublished PhD thesis. University of Western Sydney, Penrith.

Haw, J. & Dickerson, M.G. (2005). A model of the psychological process that leads to impaired control of gambling. *Electronic Journal of Gambling Issues,* (in press).

Heather, N. (1991). Impaired control over alcohol consumption. In Heather, N., Miller, W.R. & Greeley, J. (Eds), *Self-control and the Addictive Behaviours*. Sydney: Maxwell MacMillan (pp. 153–179).

Heather, N., Both, P. & Luce, A. (1998). Impaired control scale; cross-validation and relationship with treatment outcome, *Addiction*, 93(5), 761–771.

Heather, N. (2004). Personal communication.

Heather, N. & Robertson, I. (1989). *Problem Drinking* (2nd edn.). Oxford: Oxford University Press.

Heather, N., Tebbut, J.S., Mattick, R.P. & Zamir, R. (1993). Development of a scale for measuring impaired control over alcohol consumption: a preliminary report. *Journal of Studies on Alcohol*, 54, 700–709.

Hills, A., Hill, S., Mamone, N. & Dickerson, M.G. (2001). Induced mood and persistence at gaming, *Addiction*, 96(11), 1629–1638.

Hing, N. (2004). The efficacy of responsible gambling measures in NSW clubs: the gambler's perspective. *Gambling Research*, 16, 32–47.

Hudek-Knezevic, J. & Kardum, I. (2005). The structure of coping styles: a comparative study of a Croatian sample. *European Journal of Psychology* (in press).

Hurlburt, R.T., Knapp, T.J. & Knowles, S.H. (1980). Simulated slot-machine play with concurrent variable ratio and random ratio schedules of reinforcement. *Psychological Reports*, 47, 635–639.

Independent Pricing and Regulatory Tribunal (New South Wales) (IPART) (2004). *Gambling: Promoting a Culture of Responsibility.* Sydney: Independent Pricing and Regulatory Tribunal.

Inglis, K. (1985). Gambling and culture in Australia. In Caldwell, G., Sylvan, L., Dickerson, M.G. & Haig, B. (Eds), *Gambling in Australia*. Sydney: Croom Helm (pp. 5–17).

Jackson, A.C., Thomas, S.A., Thomason, N., Borrell, J., Crisp, B.R.,. Enderby, K., Fauzee, Y.H., Ho, W., Holt, T.A., Perez, E. & Smith, S. (2000). *Longitudinal Evaluation of Problem Gambling Counselling Services, Community Education Strategies and Information Products – Vol. 3: Community Education Strategies and Information Products.* Melbourne: Victorian Department of Human Services.

Jacobs, D.F. (1987). A general theory of addictions: application to theory and rehabilitation planning for pathological gamblers. In Galski, T. et al. (Eds), *The Handbook of Pathological Gambling* (pp. 169–194). Springfield Illinois: Charles C. Thomas.

Jacobs, D.F., Marston, A.R., Singer, R.D., Widaman, F., Todd, L. & Veizades, J. (1989). Children of problem gamblers. *Journal of Gambling Behavior*, 5(4), 261–268.

Janis, I. & Mann, L. (1977). *Decision-making: A Psychological Analysis of Conflict, Choice and Commitment.* New York: Academic Press.

Jellinek, E.M. (1960). *The disease concept of alcoholism.* New Haven: Hillhouse Press.

Jellinek Consultancy (1997). *The Economic and Social Impacts of Gambling in Europe.* Amsterdam: Jellinek Consultancy.

Kahneman, D. & Tversky, A. (1982). The psychology of preferences. *Scientific American*, January, 136–142.

Kallick, M., Suits, D., Dielman, T. & Hybels, J. (1976). *A survey of American gambling attitudes and behaviour.* Research Report Series. Survey Research Center, Institute for Social Research, University of Michigan.

Kamieniecki, G., Vincent, N., Allsop, S. & Lintzeris, N. (1998). Models of intervention and care for psychostimulant users. Monograph No. 32. National Drug Strategy. Canberra: Report prepared by NCETA for the Commonwealth Department of Health and Family Services.

Knapp, T. & Lech, B. (1987). Pathological gambling: a review and recommendations. *Advanced Behavior Research and Therapy*, 9, 21–49.

Korn, D., Gibbins, R. & Azmier, J. (2003). Framing public health policy towards a public health paradigm for gambling. *Journal of Gambling Studies*, 19(2), 235–256.

Kreft, I.G., de Leeuw, J. & van der Leeden, R. (1994). Review of Five Multilevel Analysis Programs: BMDP-5V, GENMOD, HLM, ML3, VARCL. *The American Statistician*, 48, 324–335.

Kuhl, J. (1992). A theory of self-regulation: action versus state orientation, self-discriminations and some applications. *Applied Psychology; An International Review*, 41(2), 97–129.

Kyngdon, A.S. (2003). *Three theories of psychological measurement in the assessment of subjective control in gambling behaviour.* Unpublished PhD Thesis. University of Western Sydney, Penrith.

Kyngdon, A.S. (2004). Comparing factor analysis and the Rasch model for ordered response categories: an investigation of the scale of gambling choices. *Journal of Applied Measurement*, 5(4), 398–418.

Kyngdon, A.S. & Dickerson, M. (1999). An experimental study of the effect of prior alcohol consumption on a simulated gambling activity. *Addiction*, 94(5), 697–707.

Kyngdon, A.S. & Dickerson, M.G. (2005). Approaches to the measurement of subjective control: an empirical study of gambling and implications for alcohol and other addictive behaviours. (*Australian Journal of Psychology*) submitted.

Ladouceur, R. & Sevigny, S. (2003). Interactive messages on video lottery terminals and persistence at gambling. *Gambling Research (Journal of the National Association for Gambling Studies, Australia)*, 15, 45–50.

Ladouceur, R. & Sevigny, S. (2005). Structural characteristics of video lotteries: effects of a "stopping" device on illusion of control and gambling persistence. *Journal of Gambling Studies* (in press).

Ladouceur, R. & Walker, M. (1996). A cognitive perspective on gambling. In: Salkovskis, P.M. (Ed.), *Trends in Cognitive-Behavioural Therapies*. New York: John Wiley & Sons (pp. 89–120).

Ladouceur, R., Gaboury, A., Bujold, A., Lachance, N. & Tremblay, S. (1991). Ecological validity of laboratory studies of videopoker gaming. *Journal of Gambling Studies*, 7, 109–116.

Ladouceur, R., Jacques, C., Giroux, I., Ferland, F. & Leblond, J. (2000). Analysis of a casino's self-exclusion program. *Journal of Gambling Studies*, 16, 453–460.

Ladouceur, R., Sylvain, C., Boutin, C., Lachance, S., Doucet, C., Leblond, J. & Jacques, C. (2001). Cognitive treatment of pathological gambling. *Journal of Nervous Mental Disease*, 189(11), 774–780.

Ladouceur, R., Sevigny, S., Blaszczynski, A., O'Connor, P. & Lavoie, C. (2003). Video lottery, winning expectancies and arousal. *Addiction*, 98, 733–738.

Langer, E.J. (1975). The illusion of control. *Journal of Personality and Social Psychology*, 32(2), 311–328.

Leary, K. & Dickerson, M.G. (1985). Levels of Arousal in High and Low Frequency Gamblers. *Behaviour Research and Therapy*, 23, 635–640.

Lejoyeux, M., Feuche, M.D., Loi, S., Solomon, J. & Ades, J. (1999). Study of impulse-control disorders among alcohol-dependent patients. *Journal of Clinical Psychiatry*, 60(5), 302–305.

Lesieur, H.R. (1984). *The Chase: Career of the Compulsive Gambler.* Massachusetts: Schenkman.

Lesieur, H. & Blume, S.B. (1987). The South Oaks Gambling Screen (the SOGS): a new instrument for the identification of pathological gamblers. *American Journal of Psychiatry*, 144, 1184–1188.

Lesieur, H. & Blume, S. (1991). Evaluation of patients treated for pathological gambling in a combined alcohol, substance abuse and pathological gambling treatment unit using the Addiction Severity Index. *British Journal of Addiction*, 86, 1017–1028.

Lesieur, H.R. & Rosenthal, R.J. (1991). *An Analysis of Pathological Gambling for the Task Force on DSM-IV. Vol.4: DSM-IV Sourcebook*. Washington DC: American Psychiatric Association.

Lesieur, H., Blume, S.B. & Zoppa, R. (1986). Alcoholism, drug abuse and gambling. *Alcoholism: Clinical and Experimental Research*, 10, 33–38.

Lesieur, H.R., Cross, J., Frank, M., Welch, M., White, C.M., Rubenstein, G., Moseley, K. & Mark, M. (1991). Gambling and pathological among university students. *Addictive Behaviors: An International Journal*, 16, 517–527.

Levitz, L.S. (1971). The experimental induction of compulsive gambling behaviours. *Dissertation Abstracts International*, 32, 1216–1217.

Lewis, D.J. & Duncan, C.P. (1958). Expectation and resistance to extinction of a lever-pulling response as a function of percentage of reinforcement and number of acquisition trials. *Journal of Experimental Psychology*, 55, 121–128.

Lieberman, D.A. (1993). *Learning: Behaviour and Cognition* (2nd edn.). California: Brooks/Cole.

Lightsey, O.R. & Hulsey, C.D. (2002). Impulsivity, coping, stress, and problem gambling among university students. *Journal of Counselling Psychology*, 49(2), 202–211.

Likert, R. (1932). A technique for the measurement of attitudes. *Archives of Psychology*, 140, 5–53.

Linden, R.D., Pope, H.G. & Jonas, J.M. (1986). Pathological gambling and major affective disorder: preliminary findings. *Journal of Clinical Psychiatry*, 134, 558–559.

Loba, P., Stewart, S.H., Klein, R.M. & Blackburn, J.R. (2001). Manipulations of the features of standard video lottery terminal (VLT) games: effects in pathological and non-pathological gamblers. *Journal of Gambling Studies*, 17, 297–321.

Loftus, G.R. & Loftus, E.K. (1983). *Mind at play*. New York: Basic Books.

Lopez Viets, V.C. & Miller, W.R. (1997). Treatment approaches for pathological gamblers. *Clinical Psychology Review*, 17(7), 689–702.

Lovibond, S.H. & Lovibond, P.F. (1995). *Manual for the Depression Anxiety Stress Scales*. Sydney, Australia: The Psychology Foundation.

Macleod, C.M. (1991). Half a century of research on the Stroop effect: an integrative review. *Psychological Review*, 109, 163–203.

Maddern, R.L. (2004). *The limit maintenance model: Temptation and restraint in gambling*. Unpublished PhD Thesis. Penrith, University of Western Sydney.

Marlatt, G.A. (1979). Alcohol use and problem drinking: a cognitive-behavioural analysis. In Kendall, P.C. & Hollon, S.D. (Eds), *Cognitive Behavioural Interventions, Theory, Research and Procedures*. London: Academic Press.

Marsh, A., Smith, L., Saunders, B. & Piek, J. (2002). The impaired control scale: confirmation and psychometric properties for social drinkers and drinkers in alcohol treatment. *Addiction*, 97, 1339–1346.

Mazur, J.-E. (1998). *Learning and Behaviour* (4th edn.). New Jersey: Prentice-Hall.

McConaghy, N., Armstrong, M., Blaszczynski, A. & Allcock, C. (1983). Controlled comparison of aversive therapy and imaginal desensitization in compulsive gambling. *British Journal of Psychiatry*, 142(April), 366–372.

McCormick, R.A. (1993). Disinhibition and negative affectivity in substance abusers with and without a gambling problem. *Addictive Behaviours*, 18(3), 331–336.

McCormick, R.A. (1994). The importance of coping skill enhancement in the treatment of the pathological gambler. *Journal of Gambling Studies*, 10, 77–86.

McCormick, R.A., Ramirez, L.F., Russo, A.M. & Taber, J.I. (1984). Affective disorders among pathological gamblers seeking treatment. *American Journal of Psychiatry*, 141(2), 215–218.

McCown, W.G. (1988). Multi-impulsive personality disorder and multiple substance abuse: evidence from members of self-help groups. *British Journal of Addiction*, 83, 431–432.

McCusker, C.G. (2001). Cognitive biases and addiction: an evolution in theory and method. *Addiction*, 96, 47–56.

McCusker, C.G. & Gettings, B. (1997). Automaticity of cognitive biases in addictive behaviours: further evidence with gamblers. *British Journal of Clinical Psychology*, 36, 543–554.

Mellers, B., Schwartz, A. & Ritov, I. (1999). Emotion-based choice. *Journal of Experimental Psychology: General*, 128, 332–345.

Michell, J. (1994). Measuring dimensions of belief by unidimensional unfolding. *Journal of Mathematical Psychology*, 38(2), 224–273.

Michell, J. (1998). Sensitivity of preferences and ratings to ordered metric structure in 90 attitudes. *Australian Journal of Psychology*, 50(3), 199–204.

Moodie, C. & Finnigan, F. (2005). A comparison of the autonomic arousal of frequent, infrequent and non-gamblers while playing fruit machines. *Addiction*, 100, 51–59.

Moos, R.H., Finney, J.W. & Cronkite, R.C. (1990). *Alcoholism Treatment: Context, Process and Outcome*. New York: Oxford University Press.

Morgan, T., Kofoed, L., Buchkoski, J. & Carr, R.D. (1996). Video lottery gambling: effects on pathological gamblers seeking treatment in South Dakota. *Journal of Gambling Studies*, 12, 451–460.

Muraven, M. & Baumeister, R.F. (2000). Self-regulation and depletion of limited resources: does self-control resemble a muscle? *Psychological Bulletin*, 126, 247–259.

Murray, J.B. (1993). Review of research on pathological gambling. *Psychological Report*, 1, 791–810.

National Gambling Impact Study Commission (NGISC) (1999). *Final Report*. Washington DC: Congress.

National Research Council (NRC) (1999). *Pathological Gambling: A Critical Review*. Washington DC: National Academy Press.

Newman, O. (1972). *Gambling: Hazard and Reward.* London: Athlone Press.

NORC (1999). *Gambling impact and behaviour study.* Final Report to the National Gambling Impact Study Commission, Washington DC.

Nova Scotia Gaming Corporation (2000). *1999–2000 Annual Report.* Halifax, NS: Author.

Nova Scotia Gaming Corporation (2003). *2002–2003 Annual Report.* Halifax, NS: Author.

Nowatzki, N.R. & Williams, R.J. (2002). Casino self-exclusion programs: a review of the issues. *International Gambling Studies,* 2, 3–26.

Oakley-Browne, M.A. & Mobberly, P.M. (2002). Interventions for pathological gambling (Cochrane Review). In *The Cochrane Library,* 1. Oxford: Update Software.

O'Connor, J.V. (2000). *An investigation of chasing behaviour and its relationship to impaired control in excessive gambling.* Unpublished PhD Thesis. Penrith, University of Western Sydney.

O'Connor, J.V. & Dickerson, M.G. (1997). Emotional and cognitive functioning in chasing gambling losses. In Coman, G., Evans, B. & Wootton, R. (Eds), *Responsible Gambling – a Future Winner.* Proceedings of the 8th National Association for Gambling Studies Conference, Melbourne. Melbourne, Australia: The National Association for Gambling Studies (pp. 280–285).

O'Connor, J.V. & Dickerson, M.G. (2003). Impaired control over gambling in gaming machine and off-course gamblers. *Addiction,* 98, 53–60.

O'Connor, J.V. & Dickerson, M.G. (2003a). Definition & measurement of chasing in off-course betting & gaming machine play. *Journal of Gambling Studies,* 19(4), 359–386.

O'Connor, J.V., Dickerson, M.G. & Phillips, M. (1995). Chasing and its relationship to impaired control over gambling. In O'Connor, J.V. (Ed.), *High Stakes in the Nineties* (2nd edn.), Proceedings of the 6th National Association for Gambling Studies Conference, Freemantle. Melbourne, Australia: The National Association for Gambling Studies (pp. 169–182).

O'Connor, J., Ashenden, R., Raven, M. & Allsop, S. (2000). *Current "Best Practice" Interventions for Gambling Problems: A Theoretical and Empirical Review.* Melbourne: Department of Human Services.

O'Connor, J., Shepherd, L., Dickerson, M.G. & Haw, J. (2005). Psychological variables contributing to impaired control of gaming machine play: empirical findings for regular gamblers. *Australian Journal of Psychology* (submitted).

Oei, T.P.S. & Raylu, N. (2003). Parental influences on offspring gambling cognitions and behaviour: preliminary findings. *Gambling Research (Journal of the National Association for Gambling Studies, Australia),* 15(2), 8–15.

O'Hara, J. (1988). *A Mugs Game: A History of Gaming and Betting in Australia.* Sydney: New South Wales University Press.

O'Hara, J. (1997). The impact of legalised off-track betting on Australian country race clubs. In Eadington, W.R. & Cornelius, J. (Eds), *Public Policy, the Social Sciences and Gambling.* Institute for the Study of Gambling and Commercial Gaming, University of Nevada (pp. 443–451).

Ohtsuka, K., Bruton, E., Borg, L. & De Luca, V. (1997). Sex differences in pathological gambling using gaming machines. *Psychological Reports,* 80, 1051–1057.

Oldman, D.J. (1978). Compulsive gamblers. *Sociological Review*, 26, 349–371.

Orford, J. (2001). *Excessive Appetites: A Psychological View of the Addictions* (2nd edn.). Wiley: Chichester.

Orford, J., Morison, V. & Somers, M. (1996). Drinking and gambling: a comparison with implications for theories of addiction. *Drug and Alcohol Review*, 15, 47–56.

Pavalko, R.M. (2001). *Problem Gambling and Its Treatment*. Springfield, Illinois: Charles C. Thomas.

Pintrich, P.R. (2000). Issues in self-regulation theory and research. *Journal of Mind and Behavior*, 21(1–2), 213–220.

Pols, R. & Hawks, D. (1991). *Is There a Safe Level of Daily Consumption of Alcohol for Men and Women?* Canberra: Australian Government Publishing Service.

Prochaska, J.O. & DiClemente C.C. (1988). Toward a comprehensive model of change. In Miller, W.R. & Heather, N. (Eds), *Treating Addictive Behaviours*. New York: Plenum Press (pp. 29–68).

Productivity Commission (1999). *Australia's gambling industries*. Report No. 10. Canberra: AusInfo.

Ramirez, L.F., McCormick, R.A., Russo, A.M. & Taber, J.I. (1983). Patterns of substance abuse in pathological gamblers undergoing treatment. *Addictive Behaviours*, 8(4), 425–428.

Raylu, N. & Oei, P.S. (2004). The Gambling Related Cognitions Scale (GRCS): development, confirmatory factor validation and psychometric properties. *Addiction*, 99, 757–769.

Reid, R.L. (1986). The psychology of the near miss. *Journal of Gambling Behavior*, 2(1), 32–39.

Reith, G. (Ed.) (2003). *Gambling: Who Wins? Who Loses?* New York: Prometheus Books.

Richards, T. & Richards, L. (1997). *Non-numerical Unstructured Data Indexing Searching and Theorising (Revision 4: NUD*IST 4) [Computer Software]*. Melbourne, Vic.: Qualitative Solutions and Research Pty. Ltd.

Ronneberg, S., Volberg, R. & Abbott, M.W. (1999). *Gambling and problem gambling in Sweden*. Report No. 2 of the National Institute of Public Health Series on Gambling. Stockholm: National Institute of Public Health.

Rosecrance, J. (1986). You can't tell the players without a scorecard: a typology of horse players. *Deviant Behavior*, 7, 77–97.

Rosenthal, R. & Lesieur, H. (1992). Self reported withdrawal symptoms and pathological gambling. *American Journal of Addictions*, 1, 150–154.

Rousseau, F.L., Valerand, R.J., Ratelle, C.F., Mageau, G.A. & Provencher, P.J. (2002). Passion and gambling: on the validation of the Gambling Passion Scale (GPS). *Journal of Gambling Studies*, 18(1), 45–65.

Rule, B.G., Nutter, R.W. & Fischer, D.G. (1971). The effect of arousal on risk-taking. *Personality: An International Journal*, 2(3), 239–247.

Russell, J.A. & Barrett, F. (1999). Core affect and prototypical emotional episodes and other things called emotions: dissecting the elephant. *Journal of Personality and Social Psychology*, 76, 805–819.

Saunders, J.B. & Aasland, O.G. (1987). *WHO Collaborative Project on the identification and treatment of persons with harmful alcohol consumption.* Report on Phase I: Development of a Screening Instrument. Geneva: World Health Organisation.

Scannell, E.D., Quirk, M.M., Smith, K., Maddern, R. & Dickerson, M. (2000). Females' coping styles and control over poker machine gambling. *Journal of Gambling Studies,* 16(4), 417–432.

Schellinck, T. & Schrans, T. (1998). *Nova Scotia video lottery players' survey.* Report for the Nova Scotia Department of Health, Halifax, Nova Scotia.

Schellinck, T. & Schrans, T. (2002). *Atlantic Lottery Corporation video lottery responsible gaming feature research.* Final Report. Halifax: Focal Research.

Schellinck, T. & Schrans, T. (2003). Surveying all adults in a household: the potential for reducing bias in prevalence estimates and the opportunity to study households with more than one problem gambler. *Gambling Research (Journal of the National Association for Gambling Studies, Australia),* 15, 51–62.

Schrans, T. & Schellinck, T. (2004). *2003 Nova Scotia Prevalence Study.* Report by Focal Research for the Department of Health Promotion, Halifax, Nova Scotia.

Schrans, T., Schellinck, T. & Walsh, G. (2000). *Department of Health Nova Scotia regular VL players follow-up study: a comparative analysis of problem development and resolution.* Report by Focal Research for the Department of Health. Halifax, Nova Scotia.

Shaffer, J., Hall, M.N. & Vander Bilt, J. (1997), *Estimating the Prevalence of Disordered Gambling Behaviour in the United States and Canada: A Meta-analysis.* Harvard: Division of Medicine, Harvard Medical School.

Sharpe, L. (2002). A reformulated cognitive – behavioural model of problem gambling: a biopsychosocial perspective. *Clinical Psychology Review,* 22(1), 1–25.

Sharpe, L. & Tarrier, N. (1993). Towards a cognitive – behavioural theory of problem gambling. *British Journal of Psychiatry,* 162, 407–412.

Sharpe, L., Tarrier, N., Schotte, D. & Spence, S.H. (1995). The role of autonomic arousal in problem gambling. *Addiction,* 90, 1529–1540.

Shepherd, L. & Dickerson, M.G. (2001). Situational coping with loss and control over gambling in poker machine players. *Australian Journal of Psychology,* 53(3), 56–89.

Simpson, T.L. & Arroyo, J.A. (1998). Coping patterns associated with alcohol-related negative consequences among college women. *Journal of Social and Clinical Psychology,* 17, 150–166.

Skinner, B.F. (1953). *Science and Human Behaviour.* New York: Free Press.

Skinner, H.A. (1979). A multivariate evaluation of the MAST. *Journal of Studies on Alcohol,* 40, 831–844.

Smart, R.G. & Ferris, J. (1996). Alcohol, drugs and gambling in the Ontario adult population. *Canadian Journal of Psychiatry,* 41, 36–45.

Sobell, M.B. & Sobell, L.C. (1976). Second year treatment outcome of alcoholics treated by individualised behaviour therapy: results. *Behaviour Research and Therapy,* 14, 195–215.

Specker, S.M., Carlson, G.A., Edmonson, K.M., Johnson, P.E. & Marcotte, M. (1996). Psychopathology in pathological gamblers seeking treatment. *Journal of Gambling Studies*, 12(1), 67–81.

Sproston, K., Erens, R. & Orford, J. (2000). *Gambling Behaviour in Britain: Results from the British Gambling Prevalence Survey*. London: National Centre for Social Research.

Spunt, B., Dupont, I., Lesieur, H., Liberty, H.J. & Hunt, D. (1998). Pathological gambling and substance misuse: a review of the literature. *Substance Use and Misuse*, 33(13), 2535–2560.

Steel, Z. & Blaszczynski, A. (1996). The factorial structure of pathological gambling. *Journal of Gambling Studies*, 12(1), 3–20.

Stinchfield, R. & Winters, K. (1996). *Treatment Effectiveness of Six State-supported Compulsive Gambling Treatment Services in Minnesota*. Minnesota: Department of Human Services.

Stockwell, T. & Gruenewald, P. (2001). Controls on the physical availability of alcohol. In Heather, N., Peters, T.J. & Stockwell T. (Eds), *International Handbook of Alcohol Dependence and Problems*. Chichester: Wiley (pp. 699–720).

Stormark, K.M., Laberg, J.C., Nordby, H. & Hugdahl, K. (2000). Alcoholics' selective attention to alcohol stimuli: automated processing? *Journal of Studies on Alcohol*, 61, 18–23.

Strickland, L.H. & Grote, F.W. (1967). Temporal presentation of winning symbols and slot machine playing. *Journal of Experimental Psychology*, 74, 10–13.

Stroop, J.R. (1935). Studies in interference in serial verbal reactions. *Journal of Experimental Psychology*, 18, 643–662.

Sweeney Research (2001). *Preliminary Review and Benchmarking of the Problem Gambling Communications Strategy*. Melbourne: Department of Human Services.

Tasmanian Gaming Commission (2004). *Australian Gambling Statistics, 2001/2–2002/3*.

Templer, D., Kaiser, G. & Siscoe, K. (1993). Correlates of pathological gambling propensity in prison inmates. *Comprehensive Psychiatry*, 34(5), 347–351.

Thomas, A. & Moore, S. (2003). The interactive effects of avoidance coping and dysphoric mood on problem gambling for female and male gamblers. *Electronic Journal of Gambling Issues*, 8, 1–18.

Thomas, S., Stoove, C., Anderson, J., Browning, C. & Kearney, E. (2000). *The impact of gaming on specific cultural groups*. Final Report. Melbourne: Victorian Casino & Gaming Authority.

Tolchard, B. & Battersby, M. (1996). The effect of treatment of pathological gamblers referred to a behavioural psychotherapy unit: outcome of three kinds of behavioural intervention. In Tolchard, B. (Ed.), *Towards 2000: The Future of Gambling*. Proceedings of the Seventh Conference of the National Association for Gambling Studies, Adelaide, Melbourne, The National Association for Gambling Studies (Australia).

Toneatto, T. (1999). Cognitive psychopathology of problem gambling. *Substance Use and Misuse*, 34, 1593–1604.

Toneatto, T., Blitz-Miller, T., Calderwood, K., Dragonetti, R. & Tsanos, A. (1997). Cognitive distortions in heavy gambling. *Journal of Gambling Studies*, 13, 253–266.

Tse, S., Brown, R. & Adams, P. (2003). *Assessment of the research on technical modifications to electronic gaming machines in NSW, Australia.* Report to the NSW Department of Gaming and Racing. NSW Government, Sydney.

Tzelgov, J., Parot, Z. & Hemit, A. (1997). Automaticity and consciousness: is perceiving the word necessary for reading it? *American Journal of Psychology*, 110, 429–446.

Victorian Casino and Gaming Authority (VCGA) (1997). *Fifth Community Patterns Survey Combined with Second Positive and Negative Perceptions of Gambling Survey.* Melbourne: Victorian Casino and Gaming Authority.

Victorian Casino and Gaming Authority (VCGA) (1999). *Australian Gambling: Comparative History and Analysis.* Melbourne: Champion Press.

Victorian Casino and Gaming Authority (VCGA) (2000). *Longitudinal Impact Study: 1999 Report.* Melbourne: Champion Press.

Viney, L., Rudd, M., Grenyer, B. and Tych, M. (1995). *Content Analysis of Scales of Psychosocial Maturity (CASPM): A Scoring Manual.* Sydney: University of Wollongong.

Viney, L., Henry, R.M. & Campbell, J. (2001). The impact of group work on adolescent offenders. *Journal of Counseling & Development*, 79(3), 373–381.

Vitaro, F., Arseneault, L. & Tremblay, R.E. (1999). Impulsivity predicts problem gambling in low SES adolescent males. *Addiction*, 94(4), 565–575.

Vogel-Sprott, M. & Fillmore, M.T. (1999). Learning theory and research. In Leonard, K.E. & Blane, H.T. (Eds), *Psychological Theories of Drinking and Alcoholism* (2nd edn.). New York: Guilford Press (pp. 292–327).

Volberg, R.A. & Abbott, M.W. (1997). Gambling and problem gambling among indigenous peoples. *Journal of Substance Use and Misuse*, 32, 1525–1538.

Volberg, R.A. & Steadman, H.J. (1988). Refining prevalence estimates of pathological gambling. *American Journal of Psychiatry*, 145, 502–505.

Wagenaar, W.A. (1988). *Paradoxes of Gambling Behaviour.* London: Lawrence Erlbaum Associates.

Wakefield, J.K. (1997). Diagnosing DSM-IV. Part 1: DSM-IV and the concept of disorder. *Behaviour Research and Therapy*, 35, 633–649.

Walker, M. (2004). The seductiveness of poker machines. *Gambling Research*, 16(2), 54–69.

Walker, M.B. (1992a). Irrational thinking among slot machine players. *Journal of Gambling Studies*, 8(3), 245–261.

Walker, M.B. (1992b). *The Psychology of Gambling.* Sydney: Pergamon Press.

Walker, M. & Dickerson, M.G. (1996). The prevalence of problem and pathological gambling: a critical analysis. *Journal of Gambling Studies*, 12, 233–249.

Walkey, F.H., Siegert, R.J., McCormick, I.A. & Taylor, A.J.W. (1987). Multiple replication of the factor structure of the inventory of socially supportive behaviours. *Journal of Community Psychology*, 15, 513–519.

Watson, D.,Wise, D., Vaidya, J. & Tellegen, A. (1999). The two general activation systems of affect: structural findings, evolutionary considerations and psychobiological evidence. *Journal of Personality and Social Psychology*, 76, 820–838.

Welte, J., Wieczorek, W., Barnes, G., Tidwell, M. -C. & Hoffman, J. (2004). The relationship of ecological and geographic factors to gambling behaviour and pathology. *Journal of Gambling Studies*, 20(4), 405–423.

Whitman-Raymond, R.G. (1988). Pathological gambling as a defence against loss. *Journal of Gambling Behavior*, 4, 99–109.

Wiebe, H.J., Single, E. & Falkowski-Ham, A. (2001). *Measuring Gambling and Problem Gambling in Ontario*. Ontario: Canadian Centre on Substance Abuse and Responsible Gambling Council.

Wilcox, M. (1983). *Wilcox Report*. Melbourne: Government of Victoria.

Winters, K.C. & Rich, T. (1998). A twin study of adult gambling behavior. *Journal of Gambling Behavior*, 14(3), 213–225.

World Health Organisation (WHO) (1982). Nomenclature and classification of drug and alcohol-related problems: a shortened version of a WHO memorandum. *British Journal of Addictions*, 77, 3–20.

World Health Organisation (WHO) (1992). *The ICD-10 Classification of Mental and Behavioural Disorders: Clinical Descriptions and Diagnostic Guidelines (10th revision)*. Geneva: World Health Organisation.

World Health Organisation (WHO) (1997). Review and evaluation of health promotion (conference working paper). *Fourth International Conference on Health Promotion*. Geneva, WHO.

Wray, I. & Dickerson, M.G. (1981). Cessation of high frequency gambling and "withdrawal" symptoms. *British Journal of Addictions*, 76, 401–405.

Wright, B.D. (1996). Comparing Rasch measurement and factor analysis. *Structural Equation Modelling*, 3(1), 3–24.

Wynne, H., Smith, G. & Jacobs, D. (1996). *Adolescent gambling and problem gambling in Alberta*. Report to the Alberta Alcohol and Drug Abuse Commission. Wynne Resources Ltd., Edmonton.

Zuckerman, M., Kuhlman, M., Joireman, J., Teta, P. & Kraft, M. (1993). A comparison of three structural models for personality: the big three, the big five and the alternative five. *Journal of Personality and Social Psychology*, 65, 757–768.

Index

Note: Page numbers in *italics* refer to figures and tables.

173